PLANS OF CA...
SPECIALTY PI...

Psychiatric/Mental Health Nursing

PLANS OF CARE FOR SPECIALTY PRACTICE

Psychiatric/Mental Health Nursing

MARGA SIMON COLER, RN, EdD, CS, CTN, FAAN

Professor
University of Conneticut
School of Nursing
Storrs, Connecticut

KAREN GOYETTE VINCENT, MS, RN, CS

Psychiatric Clinical Specialist
Olsten Kimberly Quality Care
Mental Health Division
Watertown, Massachusetts

series editor
KATHY V. GETTRUST, RN, BSN

Case Manager
Midwest Medical Home Care
Milwaukee, Wisconsin

Delmar Publishers

I(T)P™ **An International Thomson Publishing Company**

Albany NY • Bonn • Boston • Cincinnati • Detroit • London • Madrid • Melbourne
Mexico City • New York • Pacific Grove • Paris • San Francisco • Singapore • Tokyo
Toronto • Washington

NOTICE TO THE READER

Publisher does not warrant or guarantee any of the products described herein or perform any independent analysis in connection with any of the product information contained herein. Publisher does not assume, and expressly disclaims, any obligation to obtain and include information other than that provided to it by the manufacturer.

The reader is expressly warned to consider and adopt all safety precautions that might be indicated by the activities described herein and to avoid all potential hazards. By following the instructions contained herein, the reader willingly assumes all risks in connection with such instructions.

The publisher makes no representations or warranties of any kind, including but not limited to, the warranties of fitness for particular purpose or merchantability, nor are any such representations implied with respect to the material set forth herein, and the publisher takes no responsibility with respect to such material. The publisher shall not be liable for any special, consequential or exemplary damages resulting, in whole or part, from the readers' use of, or reliance upon, this material.

Cover Illustration: Jeanne Benas

Delmar Staff

Publisher: David C. Gordon
Administrative Editor: Patricia Casey
Associate Editor: Elisabeth F. Williams

Senior Project Editor: Danya M. Plotsky
Production Coordinator: Barbara A. Bullock
Art and Design Coordinator: Mary E. Siener

COPYRIGHT © 1995 by Delmar Publishers Inc.
an International Thomson Publishing Company

The ITP logo is a trademark under license.

Printed in the United States of America

For more information, contact:

Delmar Publishers Inc.
3 Columbia Circle, Box 15015
Albany, NY 12212-5015

International Thomson Publishing
Berkshire House
168-173 High Holborn
London, WC1V7AA
England

Thomas Nelson Australia
102 Dodds Street
South Melbourne 3205
Victoria, Australia

Nelson Canada
1120 Birchmont Road
Scarborough, Ontario
M1K 5G4, Canada

International Thomson Editores
Campos Eliseos 385, Piso 7
Col Polanco
11560 Mexico D F Mexico

International Thomson Publishing GmbH
Konigswinterer Str. 418
53227 Bonn
Germany

International Thomson Publishing Asia
221 Henderson Bldg. #05-10
Singapore 0315

International Thomson Publishing Japan
Kyowa Building, 3F
2-2-1 Hirakawa-cho
Chiyoda-ku, Tokyo 102
Japan

1 2 3 4 5 6 7 8 9 10 XXX 01 00 99 98 97 96 95

Library of Congress Cataloging-in-Publication Data

Coler, Marga Simon.
  Psychiatric / mental health nursing / Marga Simon Coler, Karen Goyette Vincent.
    p. cm. — (Plans of care for specialty practice)
  Includes bibliographical references and index.
  ISBN 0-8273-6102-5
  1. Psychiatric nursing. 2. Nursing care plans. I. Vincent, Karen Goyette. II. Title. III. Series.
  [DNLM: 1. Psychiatric Nursing—handbooks. 2. Patient Care Planning—handbooks.
    3. Patient Care Planning—nurse's instruction. WY 39 C689p 1995]
RC440.C566 1995
610.73'68—dc20
DNLM/DLC
for Library of Congress   94-29976
                                                                            CIP

TABLE OF CONTENTS

PREFACE

The focus for planning of patient care in mental health has become multidisciplinary. The standards of accrediting bodies such as the Joint Commission on Accreditation of Health Organizations (JCAHO) and the Clinical Practice Guidelines of the Agency for Health Care Policy and Research (AHCPR) require comprehensive care planning for patients in the community, acute care, and long-term settings, with input from all the major mental health disciplines. Yet, these standards do not necessitate that disciplines abandon their unique body of knowledge and blend into one melting pot of treatment approaches for a patient. *Plans for Care of Specialty Practice—Psychiatric/Mental Health Nursing* combines the medical diagnoses of the *Diagnostic and Statistical Manual* (DSM-IV) of the American Psychiatric Association with nursing diagnoses of the North American Nursing Diagnosis Association (NANDA) to bring psychiatric nurses into theory-based, independent nursing practice, while maintaining a collaborative relationship with other mental health care professionals.

This user-friendly guide for planning care is designed within the traditional psychiatric DSM model, thereby providing a flow from medical classification to nursing diagnoses. The book is organized into 1. sections, which list the DSM categories (i.e., Schizophrenic Disorders); and 2. chapters, which classify the individual DSM-IV diagnoses (Catatonic Schizophrenia, Undifferentiated Schizophrenia, Paranoid Schizophrenia). Each section begins with a description of the diagnostic category. It also includes the most prevalent NANDA Human Response Patterns and their universal nursing interventions under an umbrella of "nursing syndrome" (McCourt, 1990; Coler et al. in press). A psychiatric-specific nursing syndrome is a cluster of nursing diagnoses that consistently appear for patients with a specific DSM disorder. The identification of problems at the syndrome level enables the nurse to immediately begin intervening based on the standards of the profession. The practitioner recognizes, however, that individualized care goes beyond the syndrome level. Therefore, the nursing diagnoses for specific psychiatric diagnoses are identified within the individual chapters. In this way, the reader is offered two broad choices in planning care: 1. universal plans for nursing diagnoses that always occur within a broader diagnostic category (i.e., Schizophrenia) and 2. individualized plans of care with a specific DSM diagnosis (i.e., Paranoid Schizophrenia).

Nursing diagnosis-based interventions and patient outcomes are presented in nursing terminology and are supported by both nursing theory and current nursing research. The language of the text also reflects psychiatric terms used in the DSM to facilitate interdisciplinary communication from the intake interview to discharge summary, and follows it to continuity of care in the community.

Because the DSM and NANDA systems are in constant transition, and because the trend in medicine and nursing is moving toward conformity with the upcoming edition of the International Classification of Diseases (ICD), the edition numbers of the DSM and NANDA systems should be considered only as evolutionary examples.

The book is a joint venture between a clinician and academician, and every effort has been made to capitalize on this unique combination. Contributors have been selected to merge nursing education with clinical practice. While the format is simple, a variety of theoretical models have gone into the book's composition. It is aimed for the nurse practicing in hospitals, as well as in community agencies. Advanced practice nurses, educators, and students will find the book helpful in conducting care-planning conferences.

ACKNOWLEDGMENTS

The authors wish to acknowledge the task forces and individual contributors to the NANDA and DSM systems as we form another link in the chain of collaborative psychiatric practice for the well-being of the emotionally distraught patients we serve. We also thank the individual contributors to this manual who have worked diligently in combining nursing with medicine, and history with futuristic vision. We thank Kathy V. Gettrust, R.N., B.S.N. (Series Editor) for inviting us to undertake this project, Patricia E. Casey (Administrative Editor), and Elisabeth F. Williams (Editor, Health Sciences) at Delmar Publishers for their ongoing support. Lastly, without the consumer, the book would remain on the shelves. We thank you and wish you much success in your clinical endeavors. We also encourage your comments and recommendations.

CONTRIBUTORS

Joan Bavoux, MA, BA, BSN, RN, CS
Staff Nurse
Brockton/West Roxbury Veterans'
    Administration Medical Center
Brockton, MA

Lenore Utal Boles, MS, RN, CS
Nurse Counseling Group
Norwalk, CT

Marga Simon Coler, EdD, RN, CS,
    CTN
Professor
University of Connecticut
School of Nursing
Storrs, CT

Nancy B. Fisk, EdD, RN
Assistant Professor
University of Massachusetts
School of Nursing
Amherst, MA

Christine Fitzpatrick, RN, MS, CS
Director of Older Adult Program
The Boston Center
Boston, MA

Joan Norris, PhD, RN
Associate Dean
Creighton University
School of Nursing
Omaha, NE

Kathleen Owens, MS, RN, CS
Psychiatric Clinical Nurse Specialist
Brockton/West Roxbury Veterans'
Administration Medical Center
Brockton, MA

Regina Sebree, RN, MS, ARNP
Director of Nursing
Parkview Hospital of Topeka
Topeka, KS

Eileen G. Tarsky, RN
Staff Nurse
Brockton/West Roxbury Veterans'
    Administration Medical Center
Brockton, MA

Helene M. Vartelas, MSN, RN, CS
Director Hospital Services Division
Director of Nursing II
State of Connecticut
Department of Mental Health
Cedarcrest Regional Hospital
Newington, CT

Karen Goyette Vincent, MS, RN, CS
Psychiatric Clinical Specialist
Olsten Kimberly Quality Care
Mental Health Division
Watertown, MA

SERIES INTRODUCTION

Scientific and technological developments over the past several decades have revolutionized health care and care of the sick. These rapid and extensive advancements have occurred in all fields, necessitating an ever-increasing specialization of practice. For nurses to be effective in today's specialty settings, the body of clinical knowledge and skill needs to expand continually. *Plans of Care for Specialty Practice* has been written to aid the practicing nurse in meeting this challenge. The purpose of this series is to provide comprehensive, state-of-the-art plans of care and associated resource information for patient situations most commonly seen within a specialty that will serve as a standard from which care can be individualized. These plans of care are based on the profession's scientific approach to problem solving—the nursing process. Though the books are written primarily as a guide for frontline staff nurses and clinical nurse specialists practicing in specialty settings, they have application for student nurses as well.

DOCUMENTATION OF CARE

The Joint Commission on Accreditation of Healthcare Organizations (JCAHO) assumes authority for evaluating the quality and effectiveness of the practice of nursing. In 1991, the JCAHO developed its first new nursing care standards in more than a decade. One of the changes brought about by these new standards was the elimination of need for every patient to have a handwritten or computer-generated care plan in his or her chart detailing all or most of the care to be provided. The Joint Commission's standard that describes the documentation requirements stipulates that nursing assessments, identification of nursing diagnoses or patient care needs, interventions, outcomes of care, and discharge planning be permanently integrated into the clinical record. In other words, the nursing process needs to be documented. A separate care plan is no longer needed; however, planning and implementing care must continue as always, but using whatever form of documentation that has been approved by an institution. *Plans of Care for Specialty Practice* can be easily used with a wide variety of approaches to documentation of care.

ELEMENTS OF THE PLANS OF CARE

The chapter title is the presenting situation, which represents the most commonly seen conditions/disorders treated within the specialty setting. It may be a medical diagnosis (e.g., diabetes mellitus), a syndrome (e.g., acquired immunodeficiency syndrome), a surgical procedure (e.g., mastectomy), or a diagnostic/therapeutic procedure (e.g., thrombolytic therapy).

An opening paragraph provides a definition or concise overview of the presenting situation. It describes the condition and may contain pertinent physiological or psychological bases for the disorder. It is brief and not intended to replace further investigation for comprehensive understanding of the condition.

Because psychiatric nursing utilizes the *Diagnostic and Statistical Manual* of the American Psychiatric Association (1994) (DSM-IV), the sections depict the major *DSM-IV* categories, with each chapter identified under these being one of the subcategories.

This book is unique in that it identifies nursing syndromes utilizing the NANDA human response patterns as well. These syndromes permit generalized interventions that are necessary for any patient who has been given one of the identified psychiatric diagnoses within the specific major category. For example, a patient who carries the medical diagnosis Hypochondriasis, which falls within the DSM major category Somatoform Disorders, will necessarily require interventions for any patient who has been classified within that major category.

Etiologies
A listing of causative factors responsible for or contributing to the presenting situation is provided. This may include predisposing diseases, injuries or trauma, surgeries, microorganisms, genetic factors, environmental hazards, drugs, or psychosocial disorders. In presenting situations where no clear causal relationship can be established, current theories regarding the etiology may be included. For those chapters pertaining to clinical procedures, indications for the procedure are listed instead of etiologies and clinical manifestations.

Clinical Manifestations
Objective and subjective signs and symptoms that describe the particular presenting situation are included. This information is revealed as a result of a health history and physical assessment and becomes part of the data base.

Clinical/Diagnostic Findings
This component contains possible diagnostic tests and procedures that might be done to determine abnormalities associated with a particular presenting situation. The name of the diagnostic procedure and the usual abnormal findings are listed.

Nursing Diagnosis
The nursing management of the health problem commences with the planning care phase of the nursing process. This includes obtaining a comprehensive history and physical assessment, identification of the nursing diagnoses, expected outcomes, interventions, and discharge planning needs.

Diagnostic labels identified by NANDA through the Tenth National Conference in April 1992 are being used throughout this series. (Based on North American Nursing Diagnosis Association (1992). *NANDA Nursing Diagnoses: Definitions and Classification 1992-1993* (Philadelphia: NANDA).) We have also identified new diagnoses not yet on the official NANDA list. We endorse NANDA's recommendation for nurses to develop new nursing diagnoses as the need arises and we encourage nurses using this series to do the same.

"Related to" Statements
Related to statements suggest a link or connection to the nursing diagnosis and provide direction for identifying appropriate nursing interventions. They are termed contributing factors, causes, or etiologies. There is frequently more than one related to statement for a given diagnosis. For example, change in job, marital difficulties, and impending surgery may all be "related to" the patient's nursing diagnosis of anxiety.

There is disagreement at present regarding inclusion of pathophysiological/medical diagnoses in the list of related to statements. Frequently, a medical diagnosis does not provide adequate direction for nursing care. For example, the nursing diagnosis of chronic pain related to rheumatoid arthritis does not readily suggest specific nursing interventions. It is more useful for the nurse to identify specific causes of the chronic pain such as inflammations, swelling, and fatigue; these in turn suggest more specific interventions. In cases where the medical diagnosis provides the best available information, as occurs with the more medically oriented diagnoses such as decreased cardiac output or impaired gas exchange, the medical terminology is included.

Defining Characteristics
Data collection is frequently the source for identifying defining characteristics, sometimes called signs and symptoms or patient behaviors. These data, both subjective and objective, are organized into meaningful patterns and used to verify the nursing diagnosis. The most commonly seen defining characteristics for a given diagnosis are included and should not be viewed as an all-inclusive listing.

Risk Factors
Nursing diagnoses designated as high risk are supported by risk factors that direct nursing actions to reduce or prevent the problem from developing. Since these nursing diagnoses have not yet occurred, risk factors replace the listing of actual defining characteristics and related to statements.

Patient Outcomes
Patient outcomes are observable behaviors or data that measure changes in the condition of the patient after nursing treatment. They are objective indicators of progress toward prevention of the development of high-risk nursing diagnoses or resolution/modification of actual diagnoses. Like other elements of the plan of care, patient outcome statements are dynamic and must be reviewed and modified periodically as the patient progresses. Assigning realistic "target or evaluation dates" for evaluation of progress toward outcome achievement is crucial. Since there are so many considerations involved in when the outcome could be achieved (e.g., varying lengths of stay, individual patient condition), these plans of care do not include evaluation dates; the date needs to be individualized and assigned using the professional judgment and discretion of the nurse caring for the patient.

Nursing Interventions
Nursing interventions are the treatment options/actions the nurse employs to prevent, modify, or resolve the nursing diagnosis. They are driven by the related to statements and risk factors and are selected based on the outcomes to be achieved. Treatment options should be chosen only if they apply realistically to a specific patient condition. The nurse also needs to determine frequencies for each intervention based on professional judgment and individual patient need.

We have included independent and interdependent nursing interventions as they reflect current practice. We have not made a distinction between these kinds of interventions because of institutional differences and increasing independence in nursing practice. The interventions that are interdependent will require collaboration with other professionals. The nurse will need to determine when this is necessary and take appropriate action. The interventions include assessment, therapeutic, and teaching actions.

Rationales

The rationales provide scientific explanation or theoretical bases for the interventions; interventions can then be selected more intelligently and actions can be tailored to each individual's needs.

The rationales provided may be used as a quick reference for the nurse unfamiliar with the reason for a given intervention and as a tool for patient education. These rationales may include principles, theory, and/or research findings from current literature. The rationales are intended as reference information and, as such, should not be transcribed into the permanent patient record. A rationale is not provided when the intervention is self-explanatory.

Continuity of Care/Discharge Planning

Because stays in acute care hospitals are becoming shorter due to cost containment efforts, patients are frequently discharged still needing care; discharge planning is the process of anticipating and planning for needs after discharge. Effective discharge planning begins with admission and continues with ongoing assessment of the patient and family needs. Included in the continuity of care/discharge planning section are suggestions for follow-up measures, such as skilled nursing care; physical, occupational, speech, or psychiatric therapy; spiritual counseling; social service assistance; follow-up appointments; and equipment/supplies.

References

A listing of references appears at the conclusion of each plan of care or related group of plans. The purpose of the references is to cite specific work used and to specify background information or suggestions for further reading. Citings provided represent the most current nursing theory and research findings for inclusion in the plans of care. Excerpts from *Diagnostic and Statistical Manual of Mental Disorders,* 4th edition, copyright 1994, are used with permission from the American Psychiatric Association.

Clinical Clips

Interspersed throughout some of the books are brief pieces of information related to the particular specialty. The intent is to blend some concept or theory with the practical nature of the books. This information not only may enrich the nurse's knowledge base, but also may be used in the dissemination of patient education information.

A WORD ABOUT FAMILY

The authors and editors of this series recognize the vital role that family and other significant people play in the recovery of a patient. Isolation from the family unit during hospitalization may disrupt self-concept and feelings of security. Family members, or persons involved in the patient's care, must be included in the teaching to ensure that it is appropriate and will be followed. In an effort to constrain the books' size, the patient outcome, nursing intervention, and discharge planning sections usually do not include reference to the family or other significant people; however, the reader can assume that they are to be included along with the patient whenever appropriate.

ACKNOWLEDGMENTS

Any undertaking of the magnitude of this series becomes the concern of many people. I specifically thank all of the very capable nursing specialists who authored or edited the individual books. Their attention to providing state-of-the-art information in a quick, usable form offers the reader current reference information for providing excellent patient care.

The editorial staff, particularly Patricia E. Casey and Elisabeth F. Williams, and production people at Delmar Publishers have been outstanding. Their frank criticism, comments, and encouragement have improved the quality of the series.

Finally, but most importantly, I thank my husband, John, and children, Katrina and Allison, for their sacrifices and patience during yet another publishing project.

Kathy V. Gettrust
Series Editor

Delirium, Dementia, Amnestic, and Other Cognitive Disorders

Karen G. Vincent, MS, RN, CS

Delirium, Dementia, Amnestic, and Other Cognitive Disorders (DDA&C) are behavioral disorders that arise as a result of impairment in brain functioning. Whether the diagnosis is "Delirium," "Dementia," or "Alzheimer's Disease," the rationale for grouping the diagnoses in this way is their common etiology, i.e., brain pathology. Previously, diagnoses were classified according to "organic" (some underlying abnormality of the brain) vs. "functional" (nonorganic causes). The philosophy of the new *Diagnostic and Statistical Manual* (DSM-IV, 1994) is based on the increasing body of biological research in psychiatry, which acknowledges that it is impossible to isolate only a select group of diagnoses as "organic" in nature. For example, the research in "Schizophrenia" has clearly delineated areas of the brain that are dysfunctional. This new manner of classification also follows the format of the upcoming International Classification of Diseases (ICD-10).

The Nursing Syndrome for Organic Mental Disorders is represented by the human response patterns (HRP) perceiving, exchanging, and moving. The problems globally encountered by all clients with organic mental disorders can be found in the definition of these patterns.

HRP	Nursing Diagnosis	Related To
Perceiving	Sensory/perceptual alterations (specify)	Brain pathology which interferes with individual's ability to interpret and filter stimuli in the environment
Exchanging	Potential for injury	Inability to modulate and control own behaviors or objects/events in the environment which may be potentially harmful
Moving	Self-care deficit	Disorganized thought and responses that limit the ability to follow through with activities that involve steps

The Nursing Syndrome for Dementia and Delirium may be defined as the inability to perform activities of daily living due to altered interpretation of environmental stimuli and cognitive inability to follow through with established routines. Following are the generic interventions that apply to all patients with the DDA&C disorders.

Nursing Interventions	Rationales
Milieu Therapy Communication	
Keep messages short and simple; correct sensory deficits with assistive aids; redirect and refocus when confusion increases.	Brief and clear communication simplifies messages received when there is difficulty in interpreting verbal and nonverbal information.
Orient to the environment through signs, interaction with staff and family, familiar objects, or interactive groups.	Appropriate communication assists in maintaining orientation and reduces loss of ability to take action in life skills.

Nursing Interventions	Rationales
Provide consistency in schedule, i.e., eating at same time, bathing, and activities.	Consistent routines promote further orientation to time and place.

Personal Care Issues

Provide adequate nutrition and hydration, rest periods, and periodic checks of change in bowel or bladder elimination.	Due to loss of ability to process environmental and own physical cues, the patient needs assistance in basic activities of daily living.

Medication

Administer medications as prescribed for agitation and depression.	Medication can assist in regaining control of impulses, reduce agitation from psychosis, and treat depression.

Safety

Assess risk factors for falls or harming others due to loss of functioning; use environmental controls.	Safety precautions assist staff and patient to maintain safe environment yet supports maximum level of independence.

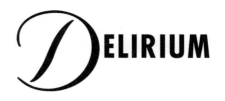
ELIRIUM

Karen G. Vincent, MS, RN, CS

Delirium is commonly defined as a disorder of attention, reflecting the patient's inability to shift attention from one set of environmental messages to another, recent memory loss, and inability to learn. The key elements that distinquish delirium from dementia are rapid onset of symptomatology and impaired level of consciousness (APA, 1993). A delirious state is reversible if the underlying etiology is treated in time.

Clinical Clip
There is a high frequency of occurrence of acute confusional states (delirium) in the hospitalized population, which often goes undetected and untreated. Recent studies show that as many as 80% of elderly patients hospitalized for an acute illness may exhibit some form of delirium. The symptom complex of delirium may be present upon admission (0.7–80%) or may develop during the hospital stay (3.3–30%) (Johnson, 1990).

ETIOLOGIES
- Medical illnesses, such as cardiac arrythmias (including myocardial infarctions); renal disease (renal failure and uremia); hepatic failure; urinary tract infections; pneumonia; postseizure states; post stroke; hypo-/hyperthyroidism; cancer; and electrolyte imbalances related to dehydration, water intoxication, malnutrition
- Acquired immunodeficiency syndrome- (AIDS-) related complex: infections involving the central nervous system, tumors, blood-borne infections; pneumocystic pneumonia; electrolyte imbalances; extreme anxiety/fear; loss of social support network; hypoglycemia; and visual losses causing changes in perception

- Drug toxicity: sleeping agents (flurazepam, triazolam, diazepam); antidepressants (amitryptyline, trazodone); cardiac medication (digitalis, inderal, channel beta blockers, antiarrthymics, diuretics); gastrointestinal (GI) medication (cimetadine); antipsychotic medication (Haloperidol; chlorpromazine, etc.); eyedrops; antihistamines; antiparkinsonian drugs (cogentin); corticosteroids; alcohol and other substances
- Psychosocial stressors: bereavement, relocation, family discord, multiple life stressors, Posttraumatic Stress Disorder, depression

CLINICAL MANIFESTATIONS
- Abrupt onset of symptoms (within hours or days)
- Short, fluctuating course; usually worse at night, in the dark, or upon awakening
- Decreased attention to environment and inability to shift attention to sets of data
- Disorganized thinking (APA, 1994)
- May exhibit
  - reduced level of consciousness
  - hallucinations, illusions, delusions
  - sleep/wake cycle disturbance
  - hyper-/hypoactivity
  - disorientation to time, place, or person
  - short-term memory loss
- Evidence of an underlying organic cause

CLINICAL/DIAGNOSTIC FINDINGS
- Mini–Mental Status Exam (confused to person, place, and time; short-term memory poor)
- Complete physical exam:
  - history of urinary tract infections, pneumonia, or history of delirium and cause
  - medication profile, which may indicate polypharmacy and its concurrent mental status changes in the elderly population
  - history of alcohol and substance abuse
  - nutrition intake
  - vitamin deficiencies or dehydration
- Complete blood work: thyroid function studies to rule out hypo-/hyperthyroidism; creatinine clearance and blood urea nitrogen (BUN) to rule out renal disease; syphillis serology; drug/toxin levels; serum B_{12} and folate
- Electrocardiogram (EKG) to rule out arrythmias
- Magnetic resonance imaging (MRI) or computerized tomography (CT) scans to rule out space-occupying lesions
- Occult blood: stool to rule out cancer of colon
- Chest x-ray to rule out pneumonia or tumor of lung
- Diagnostic ultrasound

- Neuropsychological testing to determine exact nature of cognitive changes and potential etiologies and distinquish between delirium and dementia

---
Clinical Clip

The aging process produces changes in the central cholinergic system in the brain (reducing certain neurotransmitters), which controls memory, learning, attention, and wakefulness. Anticholinergic drugs, i.e., antipsychotics and antihistamines, further reduce these chemicals and can result in delirious symptoms.

▶ NURSING DIAGNOSIS: *Sleep Pattern Disturbance*

Related To disruption in brain center which controls "wakefulness" and circadian rhythm.

Defining Characteristics
- Disturbed sleep cycle: sleeps in short periods during the night and is agitated while awake
- Interrupted sleep
- Irritability, restlessness, lethargy, listlessness, slurred or slowed speech, disorientation
- Increased confusion at night
- Fatique
- Yawning
- Possible hallucinations, delusions

Patient Outcomes
Patient will
- exhibit less anxiety and fear during the night and be able to stay in bed/room.
- nap less during the day and sleep for longer periods of time throughout the night.
- return to individual schedule of sleep and rest before onset of delirium.

Nursing Interventions	Rationales
Document sudden problems with restlessness and difficulty sleeping during the night or wandering, which are changes from usual sleep cycles.	Onset of delirium is sudden. Often, the night staff sees the first signs, via alterations in sleep cycle.

Nursing Interventions	Rationales
Assess level of consciousness during the day and at night, i.e., general orientation, state of wakefulness, sudden onset of napping during the day, and agitation.	Level of consciousness is one of the essential features of delirium.
Assess for hallucinations and paranoia during the night, which contribute to difficulty with sleep.	Environmental cues, even familiar objects, may be misinterpreted at night because low lighting can cause shadows.
Provide a quiet room and lighting, such as a night light, which will eliminate shadows.	A room free of noise from other patients, staff, or corridor sounds can decrease anxiety and promote rest and sleep. Proper lighting illuminates objects within the room.
Discourage naps during the day.	Promotes a regular sleep cycle during the night.
Ask family about bedtime routine and maintain as close as possible.	Familiar routines can be both reassuring and orienting as to the time of day.
Provide a safe environment during the night if the patient tends to get out of bed and wander.	Side rails can provide added security and a reminder not to get out of bed. If the behavior continues, however, the risk of falling over the bedrails needs to be assessed and measures used, i.e., lowering the mattress to the floor, restraint during the night, etc.
Speak in a calm, soft voice and simplify directions for tasks associated with getting ready for bed.	Emotional support and reassurance can reduce anxiety and promote sleep/rest.
Teach nursing assistive personnel and the family the cause for the confusion and reasons for difficulty with sleep/rest cycle.	Decreases the family's and personnel's anxiety and frustration about the behavior and enhances their work with them.

▶ **NURSING DIAGNOSIS:** *Altered Thought Processes*

Related To biological and psychological stressors which interfere with judgment, reasoning, memory, and attention.

Defining Characteristics
- Inaccurate interpretation of environment
- Distractability
- Hyper- or hypovigilence
- Memory deficit/problems
- Hallucinations, delusions
- Excessive indecisiveness
- Suspiciousness

Patient Outcomes
Patient will
- exhibit concentration and reality-based thinking adequate to perform activities of daily living during acute phase of illness.
- return to prior level of cognitive functioning.

Nursing Interventions	Rationales
Assess severity of confusion using mental status questionnaire.	The Mini–Mental Status Exam, a valid and reliable clinical tool consisting of three categories of information, provides baseline data about the level of confusion and can be used to assess improvement in cognitive functioning.
Evaluate for the presence of hallucinations or delusions.	Misinterpretation of cues or objects in the environment can result in delusions. Hallucinations result from underlying pathophysiology.
Assess for hearing and/or sight deficits and provide corrective devices as necessary.	Distortions in incoming cues from the environment may result from poor eyesight and/or impaired hearing. Eyeglasses and hearing aids can reduce anxiety and thus, confusion.
Utilize familiar objects to provide orientation to person, place, and time.	The presence of familiar objects brought by the family and clocks/calendars break the social isolation of confusion.
Focus on reality in brief encounters with patient.	Do not argue or agree with delusional material. If agitation or frustration increase while talking, leave the room and return with a

Nursing Interventions	Rationales
	new conversation. This technique utilizes the memory impairment.
Encourage the family to visit regularly.	Interaction with significant others will decrease anxiety and fear, provide orientation, and decrease the severity of the confusion.
Teach family and nursing assistive personnel about reality orientation techniques.	Reduces family's anxiety, which may be communicated to the patient and illicits help in providing a reality-based environment.

▶ **NURSING DIAGNOSIS:** *Impaired Verbal Communication*

Related To disorganized thought processes and symptoms of delirium.

Defining Characteristics
- Difficulty speaking or verbalizing: illogical, undirected, or unconnected speech pattern
- Difficulty forming coherent sentences
- Difficulty expressing thoughts verbally

Patient Outcomes
Patient will
- be able to communicate and receive feedback concerning basic needs during acute phase of illness.
- return to prior level of ability to communicate with others.

Nursing Interventions	Rationales
Assess for evidence of hearing impairment.	Distortion of reality and confusion can result when only portions of conversations are heard.
Assess ability to follow simple commands for tasks, such as "Pick up your toothbrush."	Behavioral rating scales clarify functional abilities.
Assess presence of pain, hunger, thirst, feelings (fear, anxiety), or need to void by using nonverbal cues.	Disorganized thinking causes inattention to both environmental stimuli and physical cues. Although unable to communicate

Nursing Interventions	Rationales
	these needs, nonverbal body language can be assessed, so interventions can be started.
Communicate in simple, concrete, and respectful manner; addressing in an adult-to-adult tone.	Communication must be simple, helpful, and constructive to assist in maintaining self-esteem.
Assist successful communication by using reflection and clarification, i.e., "I understand that you want the lights out, is that correct?"	Successful communication reduces frustration and anxiety and provides reassurance that staff is attending to their need for understanding and basic needs.
Refocus on task or conversation if patient begins to drift into delusional material.	Reorients to reality and task being performed.
Assist in utilizing nonverbal and simple communication techniques, such as nodding and yes/no answers.	By offering alternative methods for communicating needs, anxiety is reduced.
Speak in a soft and reassuring tone of voice. Assign the same staff member as often as possible.	Establishes a therapeutic alliance with the patient, which can be both reassuring and reorienting.
Teach the family and nursing assistive personnel about the effect of delirium on thinking and communication.	When family understands that difficulties are temporary, anxiety that may be conveyed to the patient is reduced.
Encourage family and other staff to speak in their usual manner.	A normal atmosphere reduces feelings of infantilization and frustration with communication difficulites and enhances return to normal ways of giving/receiving feedback.
Evaluate ability to communicate and follow simple commands as the illness is treated.	Assesses progress of treatment and return to prior level of functioning.

CONTINUITY OF CARE/DISCHARGE PLANNING
- Delirium should be resolved prior to patient returning home.
- Refer to psychosocial supports in the community (family, spouse, neighbors, friends, church, etc).

- Refer to visiting nurse agency (including home health care) for medication follow-up and assessment of psychosocial stressors.

BIBLIOGRAPHY

American Psychiatric Association (APA). (1994). *Diagnostic and statistical manual of mental disorders* (4th ed.). Washington, DC: APA.

Curl, A. (1989). Agitation and the older adult. *Journal of Psychosocial Nursing, 27*(12), 12–14.

Foreman, M., & Grabowski, R. (1992). Diagnostic dilemma: Cognitive impairment in the elderly. *Journal of Gerontological Nursing, 18*(9), 5–12.

Gettrust, K., & Brabec, P. (1992). *Nursing diagnosis in clinical practice: Guides for care planning.* Albany, NY: Delmar.

Gomez, G., & Gomez, E. (1987). Delirium. *Geriatric Nursing,* Nov./Dec., 330–332.

Jenike, M. (1989). *Geriatric psychiatry and psychopharmacology: A clinical approach.* St. Louis: Mosby-Year Book.

Mathew, L., & Sloane, P. (1991). An assessment and care planning strategy for nursing home residents with dementia. *Gerontologist, 31*(1), 128–131.

Task Force on DSM-IV, American Psychiatric Association (APA). (1993). *DSM-IV draft criteria.* Washington, DC: APA.

Wanich, C., Sullivan-Marx, E., Gottlieb, G., & Johnson, J. (1992). Functional status outcomes of a nursing intervention in hospitalized elderly. *Image: Journal of Nursing Scholarship, 24*(3), 201–207.

Wilson, H., & Kneisel, C. (1992). *Psychiatric nursing* (4th ed.). Menlo Park, CA: Addison-Wesley.

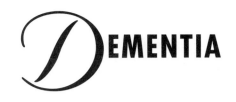

DEMENTIA

Karen G. Vincent, MS, RN, CS

Dementia is a syndrome resulting from damage to areas of the brain which control the more complex functions of memory, abstract thinking, personality, reasoning, attention, and judgment. The two most common types of dementia to be covered in this chapter will be vascular dementia and dementia of the Alzheimer type. Vascular dementia describes the etiology of the behavioral changes; there is damage in brain tissue, usually caused by arteriosclerotic changes and small strokes. The patient exhibits small steplike deteriorations in functioning. Dementia of the Alzheimer type is characterized by a steady and marked rate of decline in personality and functional abilities of the individual, resulting from changes within the brain tissue.

ETIOLOGIES

Vascular Dementia
- Arteriosclerotic changes in vessels producing three forms of lesions in the brain:
  - large cerebral cortex infarcts involving major areas of the brain
  - smaller lesions causing cavities in the subcortical areas of the brain, such as basal ganglia, thalamus, and brainstem
  - "Binswanger's disease": ischemia of the white matter of the brain causing some confusing clinical pictures

Dementia of the Alzheimer type (AD)
- Existence of neurofibrillary tangles, which are bundles of filaments wound around brain neuronal cells and neuritic plaques, which are clusters of degenerated nerve terminals. These lesions are found, upon autopsy, in large numbers in the brains of patients with AD. They interfere with functioning of the temporal and parietal lobes of the brain as well as in the hippocampus, amygdala, and subcortex.

CLINICAL MANIFESTATIONS

Vascular Dementia

- Multiple cognitive deficits characterized by
  - immediate and short-term memory loss
  - one of the following (APA, 1994): aphasia, apraxia (inability to carry out motor actions despite intact motor functions), agnosia (inability to recognize or identify familiar objects), or disturbance in the executive functions of judgment, reasoning, planning, organizing, and problem solving
- Slow progression of disease, with gradual decline in social and occupational functioning
- No correlation between cognitive deficits and central nervous system disorders, polypharmacy, or underlying delirium
- Co-occurring symptoms of cerebrovascular disease

Clinical/Diagnostic Findings

- Three key factors in assessment/diagnosis/differentiation of types of dementias: onset, duration, and progression of cognitive decline
- Tests utilized to assess for type of dementia and resulting findings:
  - Mini–Mental Status Exam—fluctuating scores on rapid assessment of cognitive function, including (a) orientation to place, person, time; (b) registration of three objects and ability to recall (counting the trials needed to total recall); (c) attention and calculation, recall, identification of objects, following three stage commands; and (d) level of consciousness
- Complete medical exam and workup:
  - computerized tomography (CT) scan—ruling out space-occupying lesions of the brain, reversible dementia states such as normal pressure hydrocephalus, and severe brain atrophy indicative of Alzheimer's disease
  - blood work—hypothyroidism or hyperthyroidism; serologic studies for syphilis (VDRL and fluorescent treponemal antibody absorption test [FTA–ABS]), testing positive; erythrocyte sedimentation rate (normal males, 0–9 mm/hr.; females, 0–20 mm/hr), any increase showing increased tissue destruction, as in collagen vascular diseases; serum levels of B_{12} lower than 130–785 pg/mL, indicator of pernicious or megaloblastic anemia
- Physical exam
- Subcortical dementias present with positive neurological signs, such as the gait in Parkinson's disease.
- Vascular dementias may also present with positive neurological signs of brain pathology (gait, hemiparesis, varying levels of aphasias, etc.)

▶ NURSING DIAGNOSIS: *Functional Incontinence*

Related To cognitive /sensory deficits and inability to connect physical sensations with action.

Defining Characteristics
• Urge to void or bladder contractions sufficiently strong to result in loss of urine before reaching appropriate receptacle

Patient Outcomes
Patient will
• exhibit a decrease in the number of episodes of incontinence.
• comply with a toileting-hygiene program.
• alert staff of need to void.

Nursing Interventions	Rationales
Assess for underlying causes of incontinence using the following eight parameters: 1. assessment of current bowel and bladder function 2. medication profile 3. evaluation and documentation of antecedents of incontinence 4. patient's ability to respond to prompts to void 5. physical exam to rule out pelvic abnormalities causing incontinence 6. assess for fecal impaction 7. urinalysis to rule out urinary tract infection 8. estimate of postvoid residual (PVR) volumes	A thorough assessment is needed to rule out physiological causes of incontinence before a behavioral program can be started.
Evaluate physical and environmental factors which may be barriers to ongoing urinary continence.	Lighting in the bathroom during the night, access to a call light and/or bed pan, toilet seat height adjusted, ability to transfer from bed to commode, picture of a toilet on the door of the bathroom, and adequate lighting to reach the bathroom will impact on toileting practices.

Nursing Interventions	Rationales
Evaluate ability to initiate voiding and follow commands.	Learning and recalling instructions will determine the success of bladder retraining programs.
Assess number of incontinence episodes in a 24-hr period.	Behavioral or prompted voiding programs are most successful when there is decreased voiding frequency and less than four episodes of incontinence in a 12-hr period.
Begin prompted voiding program: 1. Monitoring—check bed/chair and ask to verbally report wet or dry. 2. Prompting—give verbal cues to prompt patient to use toilet. 3. Praise—for maintaining continence and attempting to use toilet.	Success of this bladder-retraining program can be 75% in the nursing home population.
Establish a checking method for wetness if unable to initiate voiding.	If unable to initiate voiding, bladder training will be unsuccessful.
Limit fluids before bedtime.	This practice reduces residual bladder volume and limits urge to void during the night.
Maintain dry and clean perineal area as patient becomes more confused and less independent. Use diapers or pads and change frequently.	Cleaning the area prevents alteration in skin integrity related to wetness and immobility.
Teach staff how to implement prompted voiding technique.	Intervention will decrease number of incidents of incontinence, maintain functional level, and decrease staff time spent changing beds.
Educate family/significant others about behavioral techniques used to prevent incontinence.	Family will be able to follow through with verbal and nonverbal cues, using prompting techniques at home.
Evaluate ongoing success of retraining program and need for changes in technique.	Changes in cognition as the illness progresses may necessitate changes in bladder training/incontinence care.

▶ NURSING DIAGNOSIS: *High Risk for Constipation*

Risk Factors
- Sensory/cognitive deficits
- Immobility
- Inability to act on physical cues or sensations
- Change in appetite and/or eating patterns
- Side effects from medication
- Decreased fluid intake

Patient Outcome
Patient will exhibit normal passage of soft, formed stool on a routine basis.

Nursing Interventions	Rationales
Assess usual pattern of elimination, including timing, size, amount, ease of passage, and color.	Establish baseline data for ongoing assessment of elimination pattern.
Assess for abdominal distention or bloating, decreased bowel sounds, increased agitation, and anxiety.	Confused patients may become more agitated if they are constipated due to inability to verbalize discomfort and needs.
Evaluate medication profile.	Medications such as psychotropic or antidepressants can cause constipation.
Establish a routine time to toilet and ensure privacy.	Routine times, such as after meals when peristaltic action is increased, may help establish routine of elimination.
Assess dietary intake of fiber and fluids.	Both fiber and increased fluid intake help maintain bowel constancy. If patient wanders or paces, provide food that can be eaten while moving.
Include prunes in diet and stool softeners. Avoid use of laxatives.	Laxatives can be harsh to the intestinal mucosa and will not help to establish a pattern of bowel elimination.
If patient is mobile, encourage to walk in hall each shift.	Immobility causes constipation due to decreased peristaltic action and decreased gastric emptying.
Teach family/significant others about interventions to prevent constipation and symptoms and treatment should it occur.	Family members as direct caregivers can assist in preventing constipation.

▶ NURSING DIAGNOSIS: *High Risk for Altered Nutrition—Less Than Body Requirements*

Risk Factors
- Inability to ingest nutrients sufficient to maintain body weight
- Decreased attention span/increased confusion when accomplishing tasks, i.e., feeding self from tray containing several objects
- Reported altered taste sensation
- Lack of interest in food
- Agitation
- Poor appetite

Patient Outcomes
Patient will
- maintain body weight within normal limits.
- attend to task of feeding/eating with assistance.

Nursing Interventions	Rationales
Assess daily caloric intake from meals and snacks, including fluids.	Establishes baseline assessment of food preferences, gaps in nutrition/hydration, and teaching needs.
Monitor weight on a routine basis (weekly/daily).	Baseline weight is established as well as whether interventions to prevent weight loss are successful.
Evaluate ability to navigate process of eating.	Cognitive deficits may affect ability to follow steps of eating: identifying food, chewing, and swallowing.
Question family about food preferences.	Favorite familiar foods may encourage adequate nutritional intake.
Limit the number of plates on the meal tray or table.	Patient can focus on one task completion at a time.
Provide assistive devices to help with eating, as needed.	Neurological symptoms, such as a hemiparesis secondary to cerebrovascular accident (CVA), may hamper ability to feed self.
Provide small, frequent meals.	When tasks are simplified, patient is more likely to concentrate and complete them.

Nursing Interventions	Rationales
Facilitate patient eating in a quiet room with few distractions.	Sensory overload is reduced, ability to shift attention decreased, and likelihood of success in completing tasks increased.
Teach family/significant others techniques that will promote adequate nutrition.	Family can continue to include patient in meal time socialization and ongoing family interaction.

▶ NURSING DIAGNOSIS: *Altered Role Performance*

Related To onset of irreversible organic brain syndrome, i.e., loss of memory, inability to begin or complete tasks; disorientation to person, place, and time; and personality changes.

Defining Characteristics
- Change in others' perception of role
- Change in physical/psychological capacity to resume role
- Change in usual pattern of responsibility

Patient Outcomes
Patient will
- maintain highest level of role competency as possible during early stages of dementing illness.
- verbalize feelings about role changes resulting from cognitive decline.

Nursing Interventions	Rationales
Assess components of role loss.	Establishes baseline data of role components; expectations from others; and history of importance of role(s) in patient's life.
Assess family/significant others comprehension of severity of loss of functioning and impact on role.	Indicates stage in the family's grieving process and importance of patient in the family system.
Assist family and patient in aspects of role capacities.	Family can begin to accept the loss of various aspects of the role performance and accommodate for the person's lifestyle changes.

Nursing Interventions	Rationales
Educate about current and expected changes in functional capacity.	Anxiety is often reduced with education, i.e., changes will be expected and not catastrophic to patient and family.

▶ NURSING DIAGNOSIS: *High Risk for Caregiver Role Strain*

Risk Factors
- Severity of illness of care receiver
- Significant home care needs
- Caregiver health impairment
- Multiple caregiver roles undertaken
- Psychological/cognitive deficits of care receiver
- Marginal family functioning prior to caregiver role

Patient System Outcomes
Patient's caregivers will
- acknowledge stress involved in caring for family members.
- seek out support systems to deal with ongoing caregiving task.

Patient will
- exhibit absence of any signs of abuse/neglect in the home.

Nursing Interventions	Rationales
Assess caregiver's ability to deliver needed care to family member, i.e., physically, emotionally, and financially.	Physical limitations of the caregiver, environmental barriers within the home, financial stressors, and additional caretaking responsibilities can all impact on the caregiver's ability to sustain the constant stress of caring for a person with mental/physical impairment.
Assess level of severity of cognitive impairment/functional status of patient.	Baseline data of functional limitations of patient and extent of caregiving tasks of family are established.
Note any disturbances in family system prior to onset of dementing illness, i.e., alcohol/drug abuse, violence, or divorce.	Previously fragile family dynamics will be further stressed by a prolonged illness and early intervention may prevent abuse or neglect.

Nursing Interventions	Rationales
Assess caregiver's coping strategies.	Maladaptive coping strategies can lead to stress, burnout, anger with the affected family member, and potential abuse. Resources to help refocus the caregiver's coping abilities will assist the family unit.
Ask whether there have been any episodes of striking out/aggressive behavior.	Interventions with medication may be necessary to ensure the safety of the family members. Also, family may be helped to incorporate behavioral techniques into the care of their loved one.
Evaluate family's understanding of dementing illness.	Coping skills are compromised when there is uncertainty. Misinformation or an incorrect perception of an illness, i.e., diagnosis, treatment, and expected progression, can limit the family's ability to prepare themselves for the care. Therefore, it is important to evaluate the level of knowledge.
Teach family about illness, i.e., course and progression.	Education is known to alleviate anxiety surrounding illness. It helps the family/patient feel more in control of the disease and in anticipating increased care needs.
Encourage family/caregiver to seek external supports for help in caring for family member.	Caring for a family member with dementia is stressful; it is usually a 24-hr job. Social isolation, anger about the situation, and possible abuse/neglect may occur. Social support systems outside of the family will provide emotional outlets and validation of feelings/grief about family member's illness.
Evaluate status of ongoing caregiving during progression of patient's illness.	Be ready to act as an advocate and support system for the family, whether they are in the hospital, a nursing home, or at home. Involving the family in the care planning and care will provide needed social support.

▶ NURSING DIAGNOSIS: *Impaired Social Interaction*

Related To communication barriers and sensory/perceptual/cognitive impairment.

Defining Characteristics
- Verbalized or observed discomfort in social situations
- Verbalized or observed inability to receive or communicate a satisfying sense of belonging, caring, interest, or shared history
- Observed use of unsuccessful social interaction behaviors
- Dysfunctional interaction with peers, family, and/or others
- Family report of change in style or pattern of interaction

Patient Outcomes
Patient will
- verbalize satisfaction with activities available for socialization.
- exhibit increased appropriate interaction with family and/or peers.
- establish therapeutic alliance with staff on the unit.

Nursing Interventions	Rationales
Assess ability to interact socially with other patients during meal times, in hallway, and with roommates, visitors, or family.	A baseline picture is established of patient's ability to relate to others in social situations as well as behavioral difficulties that will guide treatment.
Observe feedback from others, verbal and nonverbal, and patient's response.	Presence and appropriateness of social skills are determined.
Evaluate patient's feelings about their quantity/quality of social interactions.	In beginning stages of a dementing illness, patients are acutely aware of their declining functioning. Encouraging verbalization of feelings may uncover underlying depression, help to begin grief process, and engage patient in treatment.
Ask family about social history, i.e., did they have many friends or were they loners?	Illustrates whether present behaviors are a change for this patient or reflect their lifestyle pattern.
Observe how patient relates to nursing staff, i.e., establishing a bond with one or more staff members.	Ability to relate to health care providers will increase likelihood of success in social skills training

Nursing Interventions	Rationales
	and increased interaction (even superficially) in groups.
Involve in activity-oriented groups, i.e., passive exercise, occupational therapy (OT), social skills training, and reminiscence groups.	Structure to the day is provided and increases social skills increased despite cognitive deficits.
Involve family members in treatment planning and activities.	Active involvement of the family in treatment will ease transition to home and social skills training used in program can be applied upon discharge.
Discharge plans should include structured day activity.	Respite for the family and social stimulation/interaction for patient are provided.

▶ NURSING DIAGNOSIS: *Hopelessness*

Related To early stage Dementia when patient is aware of decline in cognitive functioning.

Defining Characteristics
- Passivity
- Decreased verbalization
- Decreased affect or depressed mood
- Verbal cue, i.e., "I can't," sighing
- Lack of initiative
- Turning away from staff/family members
- Closing eyes, shrugging in response to speaker
- Lack of involvement in care/passively allowing care

Patient Outcomes
Patient will
- participate in self-care and pleasurable activities within limits of cognitive and/or physical deficits.
- verbalize feelings of grief/concern about declining cognitive abilities.
- maintain current social supports and add others (day care, etc.) as needed.

Nursing Interventions	Rationales
Assess for suicidal ideation.	When cognition is intact in early stages of illness and awareness is made of progressive nature of dementing illness, suicide may be considered. Hopelessness is a hallmark symptom of high risk for suicide.
Ask family/patient about activities enjoyed before onset of illness.	Baseline is established for assessing whether socializing was enjoyed prior to onset of the illness and a framework for interventions is provided.
Encourage patient to verbalize feelings of grief and concerns about future.	Verbalizing concerns provides opportunity to assess knowledge deficits, help patient work through stages of grieving, and make plans for the future, while still cognitively intact.
Progressively include in unit activities (OT, reminiscence group, problem solving).	Structured activities can support interest and opportunities for socialization.

▶ NURSING DIAGNOSIS: *Anticipatory Grieving*

Related To progressive, irreversible illness of a family member/significant other.

Defining Characteristics
- Potential loss of significant object
- Loss of ability to relate in usual manner to loved one
- Expression of distress at potential loss
- Guilt, anger, sorrow expressed by family member(s)
- Alterations in concentration, libido, sleep patterns, and eating habits
- Altered communication patterns

Patient System Outcomes
Patient system will
- verbalize feelings of loss related to family member's progressing dementia and loss of functioning.
- maintain quality relationship with family member.
- seek outside supports and social interaction during course of family member's illness.

Nursing Interventions	Rationales
Assess family's knowledge about illness, i.e., progression, course and special care needed.	Accurate knowledge about the illness, including what to expect as the dementia progresses, gives the family a greater sense of control over the illness and prevents stress-related symptoms.
Assess patient's present level of functioning.	Baseline data are established of stage of patient in the dementia process.
Evaluate family's relationship with patient in the past.	Stressors in the relationship within family in the past will be aggravated by the stress of caring for a sick family member.
Encourage verbalization of feelings of grief, loss, and anger.	Open dialogue about grief stages normalizes feelings and prevents potential abuse.
Include family in care planning for the patient.	Family's sense of control and mastery over elements of situation is enhanced, which empowers them and may reduce stress.
Encourage outside activities with support groups and friends.	Social support is a critical element in reducing caregiver role strain and helping to normalize life during the progression of a family member's disease.
Evaluate grieving process as patient's functional status declines.	Family will go through various stages of grief as patient's functional level declines; support is needed at each stage.

▶ **NURSING DIAGNOSIS:** *High Risk for Violence—Directed at Others*

Risk Factors
- Decreased impulse control due to damage to disinhibiting areas of the brain
- Increased motor activity (pacing in agitated manner)
- Past history of assault
- Goal-directed destruction of objects in environment
- Suspicion of others including paranoia, delusions, and hallucinations

- Increasing anxiety levels
- Easily upset by changes in external environment
- Inability to verbalize feelings and/or communicate in other ways

Patient Outcomes
Patient will
- not strike out at others.
- exhibit warning symptoms of increasing agitation and comply with behavioral program.

Nursing Interventions	Rationales
Observe and document events preceding a hostile or aggressive episode.	Information is provided of events in the environment that may overstimulate or contribute to the acting-out behavior.
Assess behavioral warning signals of impending violent behavior.	Baseline data are established to assess when the patient is becoming agitated and behaviors which can be warning signals to enable the staff to intervene.
Give time out in quiet environment if agitated behavior is increasing.	Environmental overstimulation from corridor sounds and other patients in close proximity may contribute to acting-out behavior.
Allow ample space for wandering or releasing excess energy as long as other patients and staff are safe.	Use of major muscle groups can help to dispel excess energy and decrease anxiety.
Approach patient from front and call out name in a low, soft voice.	Visual distortions or limited peripheral vision may impede ability to recognize caregivers and may be interpreted by patient as an assault, resulting in striking out. Approaching from a front view and calling by name will give warning of someone coming into their space.
Teach family and nursing assistive personnel about rationale for specific approaches to patients with history of striking out.	Others may take striking out or sexually provocative behavior as a personal affront that the patient has willfully thought out. Educating them about the causes for impulse acting out with dementia

Nursing Interventions	Rationales
	patients can depersonalize their therapeutic responses.
Evaluate ongoing behavior for need for psychopharmacological intervention and/or restraint.	Antipsychotics, anxiolytics, and some beta blockers have been used in successfully treating acting-out behavior in dementia patients. Use of restraints and medication needs to be based on thorough assessment and rationales.

CONTINUITY OF CARE/DISCHARGE PLANNING
- Assess family's ability to care for patient in the community.
- Refer to community-based services, i.e., visiting nurse, home health agency, and/or elder services agency in community.
- Inform family of respite or adult day health programs that may be available.
- Refer family to Alzheimer's Disease and Related Disorders Association, 70 E. Lake St., Chicago, IL 60601; phone number (800) 621-0379.

BIBLIOGRAPHY
American Psychiatric Association (APA). (1994). *Diagnostic and statistical manual of mental disorders* (4th ed.). Washington, DC: APA.

Anderson, K., Hobson, A., Steiner, P., & Rodel, B. (1992). Patients with dementia: Involving families to maximize nursing care. *Journal of Gerontological Nursing, 18*(7), 19–25.

Curl, A. (1989). Agitation and the older adult. *Journal of Psychosocial Nursing, 27*(12), 12–14.

Fulmer, T. (1989). Mistreatment of elders: Assessment, diagnosis, and intervention. *Nursing Clinics of North America, 24*(3), 707–713.

Gettrust, K., & Brabec, P. (1992). *Nursing diagnosis in clinical practice: A guide for care planning.* Albany, NY: Delmar.

Raskind, M. (1989). Psychiatric disorders in late life: Organic mental disorders. In E. Busse & D. Blazer (Eds.), *Geriatric psychiatry* (pp. 313–369). Washington, DC: American Psychiatric Press.

Sloane, P., & Mathew, L. (1991). An assessment and care planning strategy for nursing home residents with dementia. *Gerontologist, 31*(1), 128–131.

Souder, E. (1992). Diagnosing dementia: Current clinical concepts. *Journal of Gerontological Nursing, 18*(2), 5–11.

Substance-Related Disorders

Nancy B. Fisk, EdD, RN

In the *Diagnostic and Statistical Manual* (DSM-IV) (1994) most of the specific substance categories are subdivided into four conditions or phases within the substance-related disorder: Dependence, Abuse, Intoxication, and Withdrawal. For nursing, it is important to add another condition or phase to embrace nursing's broader scope of practice: abstinence/recovery. Although primary prevention interventions are beyond the scope of this volume, these should not be forgotten in the broader scope of nursing concern. Secondary prevention and relapse prevention are indeed within the purview of the abstinence/recovery status.

The DSM differentiates Substance Abuse from Substance Dependence in relative terms and by excluding the criteria for the more serious disorder (Dependence) from the definition of the less serious (Abuse), which specifies that the individual never has met the criteria for Substance Dependence for this class of substance (APA, 1994, p. 182).

Tolerance (need for increased amounts of substance to achieve same effect) and Withdrawal (characteristic Withdrawal Syndrome symptoms for the substance) are among the seven criteria for the dependence state from which three or more are definitive. If evidence of either Tolerance or Withdrawal is present, the dependence is considered physiological and must be so specified; if evidence of neither Tolerance nor Withdrawal is present, "without physiological dependence" must be specified. Thus, one can have Substance Dependence with or without physiological dependence.

Substance Intoxication is defined in DSM as "the development of a reversible substance-specific syndrome due to recent ingestion of (or exposure to) a substance" (APA, 1994, p. 183). Substance Withdrawal is "the development of a substance-specific syndrome due to the cessation of, or reduction in, the intake of a substance that the person previously used regularly. A proviso is included that the syndrome causes "clinically significant maladaptive behavioral psychological changes, or impairment in social, occupational or other important areas of functioning" associated with "intoxication" that are due to "the physiological effects of the substance on the central nervous system" (CNS) (APA, 1994, p. 183). These define medical as well as nursing phases of concern. Additionally, the nursing syndrome of Substance-Related Disorders includes the abstinence/recovery status, which is defined as voluntary substance-free periods in which use of substance of choice as well as other drugs of abuse is at zero level. It may or may not include a particular program of recovery and may or may not be permanent, given the relapsing nature of the disease of addiction. However, the long-term goal may be lifetime sobriety, and the means may be a specified program of recovery (such as Alcoholics Anonymous, Narcotics Anonymous, Cocaine Anonymous, etc.).

In many cases, a general, biologically focused nursing syndrome for this DSM category should also be considered. This may be found in the human response patterns (HRPs) exchanging and moving. These signal the nurse to be on the alert for physiological manifestations that accompany Substance-Related Disorders. The Substance-Related Disorders nursing syndrome, which might be expressed as the EM (exchanging/moving) syndrome, speaks to a state of high risk for the following nursing diagnoses:

HRP	Nursing Diagnosis	Related To
Exchanging	Constipation	Opioid use effect
	Injury (poisoning, aspiration)	Drug and/or alcohol overdose, synergism in drug interaction
	Altered Nutrition: less than body requirements	Cocaine dependence, anorexia
	Infection	Human immunodeficiency virus exposure: poor IV injection techniques, contaminated needles
	Impaired gas exchange	Chronic inhalation of toxic substances: tobacco, crack cocaine, marijuana

HRP	Nursing Diagnosis	Related To
Moving	Sleep pattern disturbance	Cocaine use effect
	Self-care deficit (bathing/hygiene)	Life-style of late stage of addictions: poor living conditions, homelessness, etc.

Nursing Interventions

Rationales

Nursing Interventions	Rationales
Assess physiological status, especially in relation to short-term pharmacological/toxic effects of specific substance(s) used, including effects of abstinence from substance.	There is a strong physiological component in substance use disorders.
Assess physiological status in relation to chronic effects of prolonged use of specific substance(s).	In settings where the primary focus of interventions is in the psychological domain and counseling is the major modality, the physiological domain may be neglected. The nurse can ensure that this will not occur.

Clinical Clip

In an attempt to avoid the reality of loss of control over alcohol, the individual chooses to remain unaware of the extent of the drinking and its negative consequences.

$\mathcal{A}$LCOHOL USE DISORDERS

Nancy B. Fisk, EdD, RN

$\mathbf{A}$lcoholism is a primary, chronic disease with genetic, psychosocial and environmental factors influencing its development and manifestations. The disease is often progressive and fatal. It is characterized by continuous or periodic impaired control over drinking, preoccupation with the drug alcohol despite adverse consequences and distortions in thinking, most notably denial. (ASAM, 1990, p. 3)

Alcohol Use Disorders can be represented by virtually all of the human response patterns because in its progression it will increasingly impoverish all human functioning. Known by many as a biopsychosocial disease, there is hardly a single nursing diagnosis that is not more probable given the presence of alcoholism in an individual; that is to say that, over time, if alcoholism is not treated and arrested, the individual will continue to deteriorate physically, mentally, psychologically, socioculturally, and spiritually. Moreover, a parallel process will occur in significant others, including, in some cases, whole family systems. Therefore, to narrow down only the most central and universal nursing diagnoses in alcohol use disorders will be a truly difficult task.

ETIOLOGIES
- Unknown
- (It is likely that abuse is on a continuum with dependence and addiction)

CLINICAL MANIFESTATIONS
(All spheres of human functioning: physical, psychological, behavioral, social, and spiritual)

- Alcohol Intoxication
- Denial
- Slurred speech
- Incoordination
- Nystagmus
- Impairment in attention or memory
- Stupor or coma (with strong odor of alcohol)
- Inappropriate or aggressive actions

33

- Mood liability
- Impaired judgment
- Impaired social or occupational functioning
- Alcohol Withdrawal
- Hyperactivity (including sweating, pulse rate greater than 100, hand tremors, psychomotor agitation)
- Anxiety

- Delirium tremens
  - nausea, vomiting or stomach "queasiness"
  - insomnia
  - transient hallucinations (auditory, visual, tactile)
  - grand mal seizures
  - illusions
  - disorientation to time, place, and person

▶ NURSING DIAGNOSIS: *Ineffective Denial*

Related To:
- Stigmatizing label of alcoholism
- Fear of Withdrawal Syndrome discomfort
- Threat of loss of alcohol for stress relief purposes

Defining Characteristics
- Denial of facts, conclusions, implications, and feelings concerning alcohol use and/or its consequences
- Refusal to seek health care
- Expression of anger if drinking or consequences of drinking are brought up
- Continuing use of alcohol despite increasing harmful consequences and losses due to drinking

Patient Outcomes
Patient will
- verbalize facts of alcohol use.
- verbalize dependence or addiction to alcohol.
- accept need for treatment.
- express feelings (anxiety, fear, etc.) in relation to abstinence and recovery.

Nursing Interventions	Rationales
Evaluate level or degree of denial.	Denial is symptomatic of the disease and can be moderate or extreme as alcoholism progresses.
Interview patient in detail about alcohol, tobacco, and other drug use. Never reinforce patient's denial by accepting false or minimizing or rationalizing statements.	Denial can be reinforced by the nurse's avoidance of open and honest communication about alcohol and other drug use.

Nursing Interventions	Rationales
Present specific facts about alcohol, alcoholism, and the family disease. Encourage questions and discussion.	Education about the facts of the disease and treatment is a critical part of recovery.
Involve family members in education with patient (or separately if family is hostile to patient).	Family and friends may also still be using denial and also require a knowledge base for their own recovery.
Collaborate with other health care team members in planning appropriate treatment referral of patient and significant other (clinical nurse specialist in addiction, if available).	A multidisciplinary approach is best in working with addicted patients as continued denial is difficult with strong concurrence among health care personnel.
Present options to patients and significant others, including a meeting with local group of Alcoholics Anonymous (AA).	

Clinical Clip

In an attempt to deny or hide the drinking problems of other family member(s), the nonalcoholic member(s) choose excessive use of ego defense mechanisms.

▶ NURSING DIAGNOSIS: *Defensive Coping*

Related To alcoholism or other drug dependence/addiction of significant other:
- parent or parents
- spouse
- son or daughter

Defining Characteristics
- Denial of obvious family/household problems
- Difficulty establishing/maintaining close relationships
- Hypersensitivity to criticism
- Projection of blame/responsibility
- Rationalization of failures and need to be perfect
- Rejection of advice/withdrawal from helping
- Superiority or rigidity of attitude toward others

Patient Outcomes

Patient will
- verbalize family/household alcohol/drug problem.
- express own feeling about this.
- understand own (inadvertent) role as codependent.
- verbalize need for ongoing treatment.

Nursing Interventions	Rationales
Assess use of defensive coping and origin of problem.	The presence of a codependency pattern needs to be determined to make appropriate referral.
Draw family-of-origin genogram and ecomap with patient and interview about use/abuse of alcohol/drugs.	Alcohol and other drug abuse patterns in past and present generations are evaluated and demonstrated to client.
Teach concept of codependency; identify codependent behavior.	Increasing awareness of own behavior helps to establish possibility of healthier choices.
Teach concepts of assertiveness and communication (e.g., using "I" statements).	Knowing how to communicate with others reduces use of nonproductive, defensive coping and provides basis for good relationships.
Refer to codependency counseling and/or Adult Children of Alcoholics (ACOA) groups.	Treatment and continuing care are necessary for personal growth and strong recovery.

▶ NURSING DIAGNOSIS: *Ineffective Family Coping (Compromised Progressing to Disabling)*

Related To family alcoholism syndrome with rigid survival roles and concomitant behavior patterns.

Defining Characteristics
- Underfunctioning chemically dependent person
- Overfunctioning partner
- Restricted communication patterns among members
- Parentified children; less than optimal care of young
- Denial of feelings (anger, anxiety, inadequacy, fear, sadness, loneliness, tension)
- Disruption of routines, schedules, and social contacts

Patient Outcomes

All or some family members will
- verbalize feelings and concerns.
- begin to communicate openly with each other.
- understand role behaviors as "family disease."
- plan and implement "family intervention."
- strive for flexibility in roles, rules, and decision making.
- utilize resources (Al-Anon, Alateen, family therapy, etc.).

Nursing Interventions	Rationales
Assess family dynamics (roles, rules, degree of impairment of coping).	Family dynamics determines the type, extent, and immediacy of help needed.
Rule out physical violence, child abuse, or neglect.	Immediate removal may be indicated in some cases.
Teach/counsel regarding family alcoholism syndrome (survival roles, behaviors, etc.).	Knowledge of dynamics and definitions as typical for this problem is vital.
Refer to clinical nurse specialist, addiction/family therapy, or other alcoholism specific therapist.	Minnesota Model (Johnson) intervention is therapy of choice for family system and individuals.
Refer to Al-Anon, Alateen, Alcoholics Anonymous, or other resources as needed.	Such resources represent ongoing support systems for the life-long recovery process.
Give therapeutic message to the nonalcoholic family members that they neither caused the drinking problem nor can be responsible for "curing" it.	Family members often feel responsible, especially the children. Alcoholic member usually reinforces the notion that it's their fault.
If alcoholic member is admitted for inpatient treatment, instruct other family members concerning early recovery issues, their roles, etc.	Information empowers family to be proactive, not reactive, and to avoid enabling behaviors.

CONTINUITY OF CARE/DISCHARGE PLANNING
- Work with discharge nurse in planning inpatient addiction treatment if needed.
- Engage in outpatient or "partial hospitalization" programs in early stages.
- Refer to AA as an ongoing part of the recovery process.
- Follow up on referrals:
  - Assist clients in making first contact.

—For continuity of care, obtain permission for release of information.
—Encourage referring person to accompany family to first/first few
sessions of AA, or to the first Al-Anon meeting.
- Arrange for ongoing therapy for patient and family.

Clinical Clip

Treatment must match patient/family needs, resources, health
insurance, etc.

BIBLIOGRAPHY

American Psychiatric Association (APA). (1994). *Diagnostic and statistical
manual of mental disorders* (4th ed.). Washington, DC: APA.

American Society of Addiction Medicine (ASAM). (1990). Disease definition
of alcoholism revised. *Addiction Review, 2*(2), 3.

Bennett, E. G., & Woolf, D. (Eds.). (1991). *Substance abuse:
Pharmacologic, developmental and clinical perspectives* (2nd ed.).
Albany, NY: Delmar.

Flavin, D. K., & Morse, R. M. (1991). What is alcoholism? Current
definitions and diagnostic criteria and their implications for treatment.
Alcohol Health and Research World, 15(4), 266–271.

Gettrust, K. V., & Brabec, P. D. (1992). *Nursing diagnosis in clinical
practice: Guides for planning care.* Albany, NY: Delmar.

Gold, M. S. (1992). Cocaine (and crack): Clinical aspects. In J. H.
Lowinson, P. Ruiz, & R. B. Millman (Eds.) & J. G. Langrod (Assoc.
Ed.), *Substance abuse: A comprehensive textbook.* (3rd ed.). Baltimore,
MD: Williams & Wilkins.

Grant, B. F., & Towle, L. H. (1991). A comparison of diagnostic criteria:
DSM-III-R, Proposed DSM-IV and Proposed ICD-10. *Alcohol Health
and Research World, 15*(4), 284–292.

Keller, M., & Doria, J. (1991). On defining alcoholism. *Alcohol, Health and
Research World, 15*(4), 253–259.

Martin, W. R., Jasinski, D. R., Haertzen, C. A., Kay, D. C., Jones, B. E.,
Mansky, P. A., & Carpenter, R. W. (1973). Methadone—a re-evaluation.
Archives of General Psychiatry, 28, 286–295.

Task Force on *DSM-IV*, American Psychiatric Association (APA). (1991).
DSM-IV options book: Work in progress. Washington, DC: APA.

$\mathcal{C}$OCAINE USE DISORDERS

Nancy B. Fisk, EdD, RN

While the Diagnostic and Statistical Manual (DSM-IV, 1994) speaks of Cocaine Dependence and Cocaine Abuse, there is much evidence that any use can be deadly. Perhaps the most respected authority on cocaine, it states that there is little difference between the "recreational user" and the "every-day addict" for cocaine has marked delusionary and addictive power. A National Helpline survey (June 1990) shows that "moderate" or "recre-ational" use is largely a matter of length of time using. Because smoking instantly delivers a higher dosage, addiction develops more rapidly. The false perception among users that cocaine is safe and nonaddictive has been enhanced by certain medical articles of the 1970s and 1980s.

The arrival of crack cocaine in the mid-1980s changed society more than any other event. The dangerous practice of freebasing, enabling users to smoke the drug and ingest much higher doses with quicker results, was no longer needed because "Crack," a lower-priced, mass-produced freebase cocaine, became available to younger users and to people of lower income.

Besides changing the sociocultural climate of use, the advent of crack affected many societal institutions, including the sports industry, workplace protocols in certain industries, the military, law enforcement systems, and even international diplomacy.

Clinical Clip

No effects are more tragic than those of perinatal cocaine use, followed closely by the strong association of cocaine use with street violence, serious injuries, and cocaine toxic psychosis.

ETIOLOGIES
(None)

CLINICAL MANIFESTATIONS

- Cerebrovascular and cardiovascular effects can occur upon single use and have been associated with sudden death [cerebrovascular accident (CVA), myocardial infarct (MI), etc.]
- Respiratory complications
- Neurotoxic effects (generalized seizures, even after a single dose)

COCAINE INTOXICATION
CLINICAL MANIFESTATIONS

- Pupillary dilation
- Perspiration or chills
- Nausea or vomiting
- Weight loss
- Psychomotor agitation or retardation
- Muscular weakness
  - dyskinesias
  - dystonia
- Respiratory depression
- Cardiac arrhythmias
- Chest pain
- Confusion
- Seizures
- Coma
- Euphoria or affective blunting
- Changes in sociability
- Hypervigilance
- Interpersonal sensitivity
- Anxiety
- Tension or anger
- Impaired judgment
- Impaired social or occupational functioning

CLINICAL/DIAGNOSTIC FINDINGS

- Tachycardia or bradycardia
- Elevated or lowered blood pressure

COCAINE WITHDRAWAL
CLINICAL MANIFESTATIONS

- Dysphoric mood

CLINICAL/DIAGNOSTIC FINDINGS

- Fatigue
- Vivid unpleasant dreams
- Insomnia or hypersomnia
- Increased appetite
- Psychomotor retardation or agitation
- Clinically significant distress
- Impairment in social, occupational, or other important areas of functioning

---
Clinical Clip

In the substitution of one element for another, safety and security of self and other are relinquished to satisfy drug craving.

▶ NURSING DIAGNOSIS: *High Risk for Trauma*

Risk Factors

- Extreme effects and side effects of "crack"/cocaine
  - danger of acute vascular effects including sudden death
  - danger of major fetal abnormalities, premature labor, etc.
  - danger operating automobiles, other moving devices under influence
- Cocaine Intoxication/Cocaine Withdrawal Symptoms
  - impaired judgment and impaired functioning
  - sensory perceptual alterations
  - disorientation, confusion
  - seizures, dyskinesias, dystonias, or coma
  - psychomotor agitation or retardation or fatigue
  - insomnia or hypersomnia

Patient Outcomes

Patient will
- understand extreme risks of cocaine use to self and others.
- verbalize desire for help to stop drug abuse.
- take measures to prevent pregnancy until drug free.
- apply safety precautions to prevent trauma to others.

Nursing Interventions	Rationales
Assess level of dependence on cocaine (frequency, dosage, route, craving patterns).	To make appropriate treatment referrals, level of dependence must be determined.
Refer to psychoeducation group (specific to substance abuse).	Such groups provide accurate information about cocaine and the disease of addiction and hope and motivation for recovery.
Provide one-to-one counseling.	A trusting relationship aids recovery.
Provide (or refer to) birth control counseling.	Fetal damage from cocaine or other drugs may be prevented with proper counseling.
Refer to 12-step programs, Alcoholics Anonymous (AA), Cocaine Anonymous (CA), and other resources as needed.	An on-going support system is helpful for life-long recovery process. It is generally believed that AA meetings are better than CA or Narcotics Anonymous (NA) for newcomers as there are more people with long-term sobriety in AA who will work well with the new person.

Nursing Interventions	Rationales
Connect patient with a temporary sponsor in AA.	Sponsorship and a home group provide a sense of belonging, which serves to anchor the newcomer to the program.
Advise that patient join a particular group fairly soon after trying out a few different meetings.	Support is imperative for life-long recovery process.
Advise abstinence from all mood-altering substances as the only safe way to remain free of the drug of choice.	Any use of psychoactive substances can trigger a "slip" or relapse into the drug of choice. Most cocaine users also use alcohol as a way to "come down" from the overstimulating effects of cocaine.

CONTINUITY OF CARE/DISCHARGE PLANNING
• Ensure that there are resources available to prevent relapse.

BIBLIOGRAPHY

American Psychiatric Association (APA). (1994). *Diagnostic and statistical manual of mental disorders* (4th ed.). Washington, DC: APA.

American Society of Addiction Medicine. (1990). Disease definition of alcoholism revised. *Addiction Review, 2*(2), 3.

Bennett, E. G., & Woolf, D. (Eds.). (1991). *Substance abuse: Pharmacologic, developmental and clinical perspectives* (2nd ed.). Albany, NY: Delmar.

Flavin, D. K., & Morse, R. M. (1991). What is alcoholism? Current definitions and diagnostic criteria and their implications for treatment. *Alcohol Health and Research World, 15*(4), 266–271.

Gettrust, K. V., & Brabec, P. D. (1992). *Nursing diagnosis in clinical practice: Guides for planning care.* Albany, NY: Delmar.

Gold, M. S. (1992). Cocaine (and crack): Clinical aspects. In J. H. Lowinson, P. Ruiz, R. B. Millman (Eds.) & J. G. Langrod (Assoc. Ed.), *Substance abuse: A comprehensive textbook* (3rd ed.). Baltimore, MD: Williams & Wilkins.

Grant, B. F., & Towle, L. H. (1991). A comparison of diagnostic criteria: DSM-III-R, Proposed DSM-IV and Proposed ICD-10. *Alcohol Health and Research World, 15*(4), 284–292.

Keller, M., & Doria, J. (1991). On defining alcoholism. *Alcohol, Health and Research World, 15*(4), 253–259.

Martin, W. R., Jasinski, D. R., Haertzen, C. A., Kay, D. C., Jones, B. E., Mansky, P. A., & Carpenter, R. W. (1973). Methadone—a re-evaluation. *Archives of General Psychiatry, 28,* 286–295.

Task Force on DSM-IV, American Psychiatric Association (APA). (1991). *DSM-IV options book: Work in progress.* Washington, DC: APA.

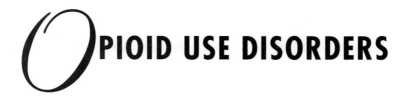

OPIOID USE DISORDERS

Nancy B. Fisk, EdD, RN

The Diagnostic and Statistical Manual (DSM-IV) defines Opioid Intoxication as "clinically significant maladaptive behavioral or psychological changes (1994, p. 249). Opioid use disorders are subcategorized As Opioid Dependence, Opioid Abuse, Opioid Intoxication, and Opioid Withdrawal. There is a strong propensity of opioids for producing physical dependence. As with other addictive diseases, the use of opioids is progressive. "Recreational" use is not acknowledged while therapeutic use for analgesia is considered potentially problematic or "at risk for" dependence/addiction.

OPIOID INTOXICATION

May or may not be as clearly observable as other types of intoxication

ETIOLOGIES
• In certain clinical conditions (i.e., chronic back pain, migraine headaches, and chronic bowel syndromes)

CLINICAL MANIFESTATIONS
• Initial euphoria followed by apathy, dysphoria, psychomotor agitation, or retardation
• Impaired judgment
• Impaired social or occupational functioning
• Pupillary constriction combined with at least one of the following:
  –drowsiness or coma
  –slurred speech
  –impairment in attention or memory

OPIOID WITHDRAWAL

May not be a highly observable phenomenon, especially if use is sporadic or less than daily

ETIOLOGIES
* Withdrawal from opioids

CLINICAL MANIFESTATIONS/DIAGNOSTIC FINDINGS
(At least three must be present)

* Dysphoric mood
* Nausea or vomiting
* Muscle aches
* Lacrimation or rhinorrhea
* Pupillary dilation

* Piloerection, or sweating
* Diarrhea
* Yawning
* Fever
* Insomnia

Clinical Clip

Methadone maintenance remains controversial in the addictions treatment field. The advantages of methadone maintenance often outweighs its disadvantages. Withdrawal from methadone is more severe and prolonged than withdrawal from heroin, which presents special concerns in females of childbearing age.

▶ NURSING DIAGNOSIS: *Chronic Low Self-Esteem*

Related To
* Age
* Sex (most apparent in women in early abstinence/recovery)
* Memory of behavior related to obtaining and/or using heroin/other drugs, which elicits shame/guilt
* Abusive, rejecting, or hypercritical parent(s)

Defining Characteristics
* Negative perception of self
  −evaluates self as unable to deal with events
  −exaggerates negative feedback about self
  −expression of shame or guilt about past behavior
  −self-negating verbalizations despite present sobriety
* Hypercritical, abusive, or neglectful mate
* Powerlessness

Patient Outcomes

Patient will
- begin to accept and perceive self as a person of value/worth.
- express feelings of adequacy and competence.
- evaluate self realistically (strengths and limitations).
- engage in self-improvement activity, setting realistic goals.

Nursing Interventions	Rationales
Assess and validate problem origin and current contributing factors.	Baseline information is essential for collaborative solving of problem.
Demonstrate acceptance of patient as a unique and worthwhile person.	Personal dignity is thus respected by another as model for self-respect.
Assist patient in identifying strengths and reinforce these.	Reality-based data need to be identified for incorporation into own self-worth.
Encourage patient to begin and continue the steps of the Alcoholics Anonymous (AA) program.	The AA steps provide for taking personal moral inventory and sharing with a trusted person in cathartic process. Making amends to individuals harmed serves to clear the slate.

Clinical Clip

Because of the priority that drug seeking has in a substance abuser's life, important relationships may be lost or altered.

▶ NURSING DIAGNOSIS: *High Risk for Altered Parenting*

Risk Factors
- Time and attention devoted to obtaining drug supply may cause lapses in child care
- Effects of drug intoxication: drowsiness or coma, impairment in attention or memory
- Effects of drug withdrawal: dysphoric mood, flulike symptoms
- Ineffective role model (perhaps)
- Inappropriate caretaking behaviors (feeding, safety, etc.)
- Child abuse, neglect, or abandonment

- Inconsistent discipline (overpermissive or demanding)
- Multiple caretakers (in drug subcultures) (perhaps)

Patient Outcomes
Patient will
- understand dangers to self and child/children of continued use of opioids.
- seek out treatment: abstinence focused or methadone maintenance program.
- work out contractual agreement for alternative child care if necessary for children's well-being.

Nursing Interventions	Rationales
Assess degree of risk to children (neglect, abuse, etc.).	Not every substance-abusing individual is a neglectful or abusive parent; however, it is essential that alternative care be provided if neglect or abuse is present.
Provide support systems which enable children to safely remain with parent(s).	It is not always necessary to remove child from parent's home if adequate help is provided through family or community resources.
Teach/counsel about disease of addiction and recovery process.	Knowledge may empower patient to consider treatment and recovery.
Refer to addiction-specific psycho-educational group.	Psychoeducational groups can provide group support and confrontation of denial.
Refer to methadone maintenance program if available.	This may be the best recourse where previous attempts at recovery have failed or where client expresses inability to cease drug use. Children will achieve greater independence with each passing year.
Provide or refer to birth control information.	This helps to prevent further pregnancies while mother is actively using drugs or at risk for relapse.
Guide parent(s) concerning developmental needs of child.	Age-appropriate anticipatory guidance will enhance child's psychological growth and development.
Initiate regular case conferencing.	Interteam collaboration maintains consistency of interventions.

— **Clinical Clip** —

Because of the toxic effects of alcohol and/or other drugs on the brain, reversible or irreversible brain syndromes occur with variable effects of cognitive patterns.

▶ NURSING DIAGNOSIS: *Altered Thought Processes*

Related To:
- Direct alcohol/other drug toxicity while under influence
- Acute withdrawal syndromes, e.g., delirium tremens
- Long-term effects of alcohol/drugs on central nervous system (CNS), leading to brain damage (e.g., Korsakoff syndrome)

Defining Characteristics
- Confusion, slowed thinking
- Delusions, hallucinations
- Grandiosity, inaccurate perception of self
- Hyper- or hypovigilance, suspiciousness
- Inaccurate interpretation of environment
- Short-term memory deficit
- Learning inability for new information

Patient Outcomes
Patient will
- safely detoxify from alcohol and all other drugs.
- arrest brain damage (if present) at present level.
- restore physical health and nutrition status to optimal level possible.
- remain substance free in sheltered environment.

Nursing Interventions	Rationales
Assess and monitor changes in thought processes in relation to degree of intoxication or state of withdrawal or irreversibility.	Cause/effect patterns are determined as basis for appropriate treatment or referral for definitive care.
Medicate as per protocols for detoxification for substances used and estimated blood levels based on history and physical findings.	Medication helps to avoid or eliminate severe, life-threatening withdrawal syndromes.
Protect from physical harm to self or others.	Inaccurate perception of reality may cause patient to react defensively or violently.

Nursing Interventions	Rationales
Refer patient to appropriate long-term care in program tailored to needs of chronic, late-stage alcoholic and drug-addicted individuals, e.g., halfway house.	This may be the only humane way to keep person from continued deterioration and self-annihilation.
Arrange case conference with other nurses, physician, social worker, family members (if involved), and other social service providers.	Multidisciplinary and network approaches are most productive by bringing all resources together to consider all possible aftercare options.
Keep aware that no case can ever be determined to be completely hopeless and no health care person should refuse to apply effort toward recovery.	Recovery has happened even when the outlook appeared to be zero in terms of hope.

CONTINUITY OF CARE/DISCHARGE PLANNING
- Monitor progress for sake of safety of children, especially if patient continues actively to use street drugs.
- Support and encourage patient if on methadone or in recovery because of low self-esteem and feelings of incompetence in parenting, etc.
- Initiate interdisciplinary collaboration.
- Refer to sheltered environment (i.e., halfway house or a long-term rehabilitation facility) for patients who continue to actively abuse alcohol and other drugs.
- Refer to a shelter for homeless persons as a final option.

BIBLIOGRAPHY
American Psychiatric Association (APA). (1994). *Diagnostic and statistical manual of mental disorders* (4th ed.). Washington, DC: APA.

American Society of Addiction Medicine. (1990). Disease definition of alcoholism revised. *Addiction Review, 2*(2), 3.

Bennett, E. G., & Woolf, D. (Eds.). (1991). *Substance abuse: Pharmacologic, developmental and clinical perspectives* (2nd ed.). Albany, NY: Delmar.

Flavin, D. K., & Morse, R. M. (1991). What is alcoholism? Current definitions and diagnostic criteria and their implications for treatment. *Alcohol Health and Research World, 15*(4), 266–271.

Gettrust, K. V., & Brabec, P. D. (1992). *Nursing diagnosis in clinical practice: Guides for planning care.* Albany, NY: Delmar.

Gold, M. S. (1992). Cocaine (and crack): Clinical aspects. In J. H. Lowinson, P. Ruiz, R. B. Millman (Eds.) & J. G. Langrod (Assoc. Ed.), *Substance abuse: A comprehensive textbook* (3rd ed.). Baltimore, MD: Williams & Wilkins.

Grant, B. F., & Towle, L. H. (1991). A comparison of diagnostic criteria: DSM-III-R, Proposed DSM-IV and Proposed ICD-10. *Alcohol Health and Research World, 15*(4), 284–292.

Keller, M., & Doria, J. (1991). On defining alcoholism. *Alcohol, Health and Research World, 15*(4), 253–259.

Martin, W. R., Jasinski, D. R., Haertzen, C. A., Kay, D. C., Jones, B. E., Mansky, P. A., & Carpenter, R. W. (1973). Methadone—a re-evaluation. *Archives of General Psychiatry, 28,* 286–295.

Task Force on DSM-IV, American Psychiatric Association (APA). (1991). *DSM-IV options book: Work in progress.* Washington, DC: APA.

Schizophrenia

Kathleen Owens, MSN, RN, CS

The nursing syndrome for schizophrenia is represented by the human response patterns knowing, relating, choosing, feeling, and moving. It illustrates the profound effect of this illness on all areas of functioning.

HRP	Nursing Diagnosis	Related To
Knowing	Altered thought processes	Biochemical and structural changes in the brain
Relating	Impaired social interaction	Altered sense or interpretation of reality; difficulty with social skills
Choosing	Ineffective individual coping	Poor cognitive skills
Feeling	High risk for violence	Symptoms of schizophrenia leading to paranoia or panic around others
Moving	Self-care deficit	Altered relationship to body inattention to environment
	Altered health maintenance	Cognitive deficits

$\mathcal{S}$CHIZOPHRENIA

Kathleen Owens, MSN, RN, CS

$\mathcal{S}$chizophrenia describes groupings of psychiatric symptoms characterized by disturbances in thought processes, behavior, and emotions. While there are variations within and between patients, Schizophrenia is generally a chronic illness that results in a decreased level of functioning or an inability to attain an expected level of functioning. Schizophrenia is divided into five types: Paranoia, Catatonic, Disorganized, Undifferentiated, and Residual.

ETIOLOGIES
- Unknown
- Possible genetic susceptibility
- Illness may not be precipitated unless other stressors come in to play
- Equal occurrence in males and females

CLINICAL MANIFESTATIONS
Generally Applicable to All Types:
- A prodromal period where there is a change in usual behavior, such as increased social isolation, the appearance of "odd" or eccentric behavior, and a decrease in the level of daily functioning
- An active phase characterized by the presence or absence of positive and negative symptoms and the identification of a particular subtype of the illness
  - positive symptoms: delusions, hallucinations, disorganized speech
  - negative symptoms: flat affect, avolition, alogia, anhedonia

Behavioral Manifestations of Specific Subtypes:
- Paranoid Schizophrenia
  - preoccupation with systematized delusions or auditory hallucinations related to a single theme
  - guarded
  - suspiciousness, leading to risk for violence

- Catatonic Schizophrenia
  - catatonic stupor
  - catatonic negativism
  - catatonic rigidity
  - catatonic excitement
  - catatonic posturing (immobility, standing or sitting in one position for hours)
- Disorganized Schizophrenia
  - incoherence, marked loosening of associations, or grossly disorganized behavior
  - flat or grossly inappropriate affect
  - inability to problem solve
  - unable to perform activities of daily living (ADL)
  - inability to communicate
- Undifferentiated Schizophrenia
  - delusions
  - hallucinations
  - incoherence
  - grossly disorganized behavior
- Residual Schizophrenia
  - absence of prominent delusions, hallucinations, incoherence, or grossly disturbed speech
  - evidence of problems with thinking, behavior, emotions, or socialization
  - illogical thinking
  - emotional blunting
  - mild loosening of associations

CLINICAL/DIAGNOSTIC FINDINGS
- Present for treatment with severe psychotic symptoms after a prodromal period where behavior has been described as withdrawn or unusual or there has been some impairment in functioning
- Physical exam and computerized tomography (CT) scans to rule out brain lesions and studies to rule out organic causes of psychosis, i.e., medication and underlying medical conditions
- Diagnosis is based on the personal and family history and current symptomatology
- Psychological testing to rule out organicity

▶ NURSING DIAGNOSIS: *Altered Thought Processes*

Related To
- Schizophrenia
- Vulnerability to increased stress levels

Defining Characteristics
- Inappropriate, non-reality-based thinking
- Inaccurate interpretation of the environment

Patient Outcomes

Patient will

- verbalize or demonstrate a decrease in distress related to delusions, hallucinations, or other cognitive distortions.
- be oriented to person, place, time, and self.
- be able to participate in therapeutic activities.
- verbalize one way of coping with distressing hallucinations.

Nursing Interventions	Rationales
Assess and document mental status and identify how symptoms interfere with daily functioning skills.	This allows for individualized care based upon the most dysfunctional symptoms.
Provide a reality-oriented milieu.	Such an atmosphere helps correct distortions and misperceptions of the environment (people, events, objects, etc.).
Be attentive to the themes that may increase hallucinations or delusional talk.	Non-reality-based thinking may increase when anxiety level increases.
Be attentive to the themes from hallucinations, delusions, and other cognitive distortions.	Concerns or fears may be expressed as metaphors through these methods (e.g., safety, need to escape, fear of others, sadness.)
Provide a safe environment.	Distortions in thinking may place patients or others at risk for injury, i.e., command hallucinations to harm themselves or others or delusional belief that they can act out a dangerous behavior safely, e.g., "I can fly."
Teach how to cope with distressing hallucinations.	Techniques such as humming, using a radio, or telling the voices to "go away" can be used for symptom relief.

▶ NURSING DIAGNOSIS: *Impaired Social Interaction*

Related To

- Cognitive impairment
- Bizarre and socially inappropriate behavior
- Fear of others

Defining Characteristics
- Verbalized or observed discomfort in social situations
- Verbalized or observed inability to receive or communicate a satisfying sense of belonging, caring, interest, or shared history
- Observed use of unsuccessful social interaction behaviors
- Dysfunctional interaction with peers, family, and/or others

Patient Outcomes
Patient will
- demonstrate how to make requests in a socially acceptable manner.
- exhibit less discomfort in previously stressful social situations.
- be able to identify types of social situations which feel more comfortable.
- exhibit less dysfunctional interaction with peers, family, and/or others.

Nursing Interventions	Rationales
Assess and document past experiences and patterns of social activity and interaction.	Previous level of functioning and the types of activities enjoyed are identified.
Assess current strengths and problem areas regarding social interactions.	Areas of strength to reinforce and build upon are identified as well as problem areas that can be improved.
Identify, with the patient, goals for increased social interaction.	Compliance is increased when the patient is part of the decision-making process.
Support and reinforce efforts and successes in social interactions. (Be specific regarding the situations to be reinforced.)	Positive reinforcement, even for slight movement toward the expected behavior change, is very reinforcing and encouraging when patients are trying to master a new behavior.
Teach essential components of appropriate social interaction. Begin with simple steps of social interaction, such as making eye contact during conversation, productive patterns of speech, and how to relate the message.	Addresses gaps in knowledge of social skills.
Provide emotional support as patient tries to reach goals.	Patients often have low self-esteem and may be very discouraged by their own performance or the reactions of others to their efforts to

Nursing Interventions	Rationales
	socialize and communicate. Empathetic listening and support can enhance self-esteem by allowing verbalization without criticism while learning a new behavior.
Provide a group situation to improve social skills.	Provides an opportunity to practice skills for social interaction in a less threatening and more supportive environment.
Evaluate the care plan as needed, and at regular intervals, to ensure that the direction and method of treatment is appropriate.	This ensures that the goals are neither too advanced nor too basic for the patient's need and that the opportunities for skill development match the need.

▶ NURSING DIAGNOSIS: *Ineffective Individual Coping*

Related To
- Personal vulnerability
- Cognitive deficits
- Coexisting substance abuse disorder

Defining Characteristics
- Inability to problem solve
- Alteration in social participation
- Destructive behavior toward self or others

Patient Outcomes
Patient will
- learn steps in the problem-solving process.
- be able to generalize these steps to other situations in own life.
- identify situations or events that may be high risk for stress.
- develop alternative ways of coping with the high-risk situations that may increase symptoms.

Nursing Interventions	Rationales
Assess and document current coping mechanisms.	Strengths and problem areas are identified and staff allowed to set realistic expectations for behavior.

Nursing Interventions	Rationales
Help patients identify high-risk situations and develop alternate ways of coping.	When situations that may precipitate an increase in symptoms are identified, strategies to avoid or decrease the stimulus or resulting anxiety may be developed.
Teach steps in problem-solving process.	A step-by-step structure is helpful for people whose thoughts are disorganized.
Provide practice situations to use new problem-solving skills.	Using skills in "field test" situations helps build confidence and provides opportunities to generalize the use of the skills.

▶ NURSING DIAGNOSIS: *High Risk for Violence*

Risk Factors
- Poor impulse control
- Command hallucinations to harm others or protect oneself
- Fear/panic when approached by others
- Decreased tolerance of environmental stimuli
- Body language (clenched fist, tense facial expression, rigid posture, taughtness indicating effort to control)
- Hostile, threatening verbalizations
- Increased motor activity (pacing, excitement, irritability, agitation)
- Overt aggressive acts
- Suspicion of others
- Delusion
- Hallucinations

Patient Outcomes
Patient will
- not injure himself/herself or others.
- communicate with staff when feeling distressed and at risk for losing control.
- identify stressors (internal or external) which increase risk for acting aggressively.
- identify alternative ways of coping with the stressors.
- report feeling of increased self-esteem when using more acceptable coping responses.

Nursing Interventions	Rationales
Assess and document past history of violence and current risk factors.	Care is planned to modify risk factors that would place anyone (patients, staff, or visitors) in any danger.
Design a contract to seek out staff when patient begins to experience precursors to violence.	A contract helps give the patient control and responsibility in avoiding a possible violent outburst and provides an opportunity to learn new ways of coping.
Provide a safe environment.	It is important for paranoid, fearful patients with cognitive impairments to have sufficient personal space, areas with decreased stimulation, and staff sensitive to their special needs.
Provide intervention based on past history and current presenting symptoms.	Interventions are matched to needs and may include empathetic listening, cognitive restructuring, emotional support, stress management techniques, limit setting, and/or physical containment.
Teach how to identify stressors for risk of loss of control and strategies for coping.	Self-mastery and self-esteem are increased when stressor(s) can be identified and understood and changes made in behavior.
Discuss the possible risk factors for violence in the community and strategies for safety.	The use of learned coping mechanisms and self-control after discharge are encouraged.
Include the family or significant other in teaching about safety.	Patients and others are encouraged to use alternatives to possible violence.

▶ NURSING DIAGNOSIS: *Altered Health Maintenance*

Related To:
- Significant alteration in communication skills
- Lack of ability to make deliberate and thoughtful judgments
- Perceptual/cognitive impairment

Defining Characteristics
- Demonstrated lack of knowledge regarding basic health practices
- Demonstrated lack of adaptive behaviors to internal/external environmental changes
- Reported or observed inability to take responsibility for meeting basic health practices in any or all functional pattern areas
- Lack of ability to make deliberate and thoughtful judgments
- Perceptual/cognitive impairment

Patient Outcomes
Patient will
- verbalize an understanding of why medication is needed even when outside the hospital.
- be able to describe symptoms and the effects of medication.
- be able to describe common side effects of medication and what to do if experienced.
- be able to verbalize the reasons for continuing in treatment when leaving the hospital.

Nursing Interventions	Rationales
Assess and document knowledge and beliefs regarding Schizophrenia, the use of medication, and the treatment resources.	Misinformation and distortions in understanding of Schizophrenia and its treatment need to be addressed early to promote active participation in and compliance with treatment.
Help link symptom reduction with the use of medication.	Education relates treatment to symptom control and may increase compliance with medication.
Teach about precautions and medication effects and how to best respond to or manage them.	Some of the distressing side effects and risks of medication, what they mean, and what may help are acknowledged. This allows for a risk/benefit discussion which may increase participation in treatment, including continuing to take medication and responding to problems in a more knowledgeable manner.
Develop the discharge plan with the patient/family to elicit support for medication use and follow-up care.	Supportive involvement of the family/significant other may increase the patient's compliance with treatment.

► NURSING DIAGNOSIS: *Bathing/Hygiene Self-Care Deficit*

Related To perceptual/cognitive impairment.

Defining Characteristics
* Inability to wash body or body parts
* Inability to obtain or get to water source
* Inability to regulate temperature flow

Patient Outcomes
Patient will
* maintain or increase bathing/hygiene skills.
* complete bathing/hygiene regimen at optimal level of independence.
* have maintained bathing/hygiene at optimal level for prior to discharge.

Nursing Interventions	Rationales
Assess and document current level of functioning and possible reasons for the deficits.	A foundation of capabilities is established and problem areas identified which may include skill deficits (i.e., uses water but will not use soap or a washcloth; washes correctly but will not change clothes) as well as the etiology of the behavior (i.e., unable to organize bathing steps; delusional about changing clothing).
Individualize a care plan to support current level of functioning and increase independence in completing the bathing/hygiene regime. Develop a system for rating how well the patient does each day in achieving the goals and the type of reinforcement that is effective.	Bathing and hygiene levels are maintained while promoting increasing independence for self-care. This may start with physical assistance and move to minimal or absent verbal prompting.
Teach about social and health benefits of bathing and hygiene.	An opportunity is provided to reinforce the care plan and address any unique concerns.

► NURSING DIAGNOSIS: *Dressing/Grooming Self-Care Deficit*

Related To cognitive/perceptual impairment.

Defining Characteristic

- Inability to maintain appearance at a satisfactory level

Patient Outcomes

Patient will
- dress appropriately for weather conditions.
- change clothes at regular intervals.
- complete grooming activities independently.
- acknowledge increased self-esteem when dressed and groomed appropriately.

Nursing Interventions	Rationales
Assess and document the patient's current strengths and deficits in these areas.	Positive skills need to be maintained while addressing problems.
Assess any special meanings that prompt dressing or grooming in a particular manner.	It is important to know any special meanings attached to dressing/grooming behavior that is problematic.
Ensure easy access to clothing, toilet articles, mirror, and other dressing and grooming needs.	Patients with thought disorders can be easily overwhelmed if preparatory activity is too complex; they also need sufficient time to complete the activity at their own pace.
Provide support needed to complete the grooming/hygiene activity.	Physical assistance may be required when first admitted or when more psychotic. Verbal direction should be clear, concise, simple, and repeated often.
Establish a group specifically to address dressing/grooming deficits.	This decreases the intensity of one-on-one interaction, which may be uncomfortable, and provides a supportive group of peers to enhance both socialization opportunities and learning.
Educate about appropriate dress for weather conditions.	Patients may be less sensitive to temperature changes because of their illness and/or the effects of medication and may be at risk for heat or cold injury.

CONTINUITY OF CARE/DISCHARGE PLANNING

- Encourage involvement in day hospital and day treatment programs.
- Provide instructions for continued individual therapy and medication use.
- Help to establish a supportive living arrangement and sheltered work environment.
- Refer to community support programs, visiting nurse associations, and family support groups.

BIBLIOGRAPHY

Cooper, K. H. (1984). Territorial behavior among the institutionalized: A nursing perspective. *Journal of Psychosocial Nursing, 22*(12), 6–11.

Corrigan, P. W., & Storzbach, D. M. (1993). Behavioral interventions for alleviating psychotic symptoms. *Hospital and Community Psychiatry, 44*(4), 341–346.

Hamera, E. et al. (1992). Symptom monitoring in schizophrenia: Potential for enhancing self-care. *Archives of Psychiatric Nursing, 6*(6), 324–330.

Harmon, R. B., & Tratnack, S. A. (1992). Teaching hospitalized patients with serious, persistent mental illness. *Journal of Psychosocial Nursing, 30*(7), 33–36.

Sclafani, M. (1986). Violence and behavior control. *Journal of Psychosocial Nursing, 24*(11), 8–13.

Mood Disorders

Karen G. Vincent, MS, RN, CS

The term *mood* refers to an individual's inner experience of emotions and the behavioral expression of those emotions. The psychiatric disorders characterized by uncontrolled fluctuations in "moods" or "affect" are broadly labeled mood disorders. They include the extremes of the emotional spectrum: the highs of manic behavior in bipolar disease to the utter despair experienced with major depression. The diagnoses covered in this chapter are specifically the Bipolar Disorders of Manic Depression and Cyclothymia and the unipolar depressive disorders, including Major Depression and Dysthymia.

The nursing syndrome for Mood Disorders is represented by the human response patterns (HRPs) moving, exchanging, relating, choosing, and knowing.

HRP	Nursing Diagnosis	Related To
Moving	Sleep pattern disturbance	Disruption of biological regulating mechanisms for sleep
Relating	Altered sexuality patterns	Heightened or decreased libido resulting from biochemical/neurological imbalances
Choosing	Ineffective individual coping	Constant shifting of mood and/or thought processes, which interferes with establishing effective adaptive coping strategies
Knowing	Altered thought processes	Rapid, racing thoughts and inability to attend to tasks; interferes with judgment and decision-making processes
Exchanging	High risk for altered nutrition	Activity level(s) which interfere with regular eating patterns

Nursing Interventions

Sleep Pattern Disturbance

Reduce "naps" during the day; establish a consistent bed time schedule; decrease stimuli in the environment to enhance sleeping.

Use as-needed antianxiety or antipsychotic medication if sleeping is consistently difficult.

Gently but firmly put patient back to bed when he or she attempts to arise in middle of the night.

Rationales

The Mood Disorders interrupt regular sleep/rest patterns. Thus, interventions are needed to promote a quiet environment to encourage sleep.

Psychopharmacological agents are helpful in decreasing anxiety and/or agitation and promoting sleep.

Regular sleep patterns are established and anxiety/agitation may be decreased. Stimulating activities are avoided before or during appropriate sleep times.

Nursing Interventions	**Rationales**
Altered Sexuality Patterns	
Assess changes in routine sexuality patterns, i.e., hyper- or hyposexual behaviors.	Baseline behavior is established before manic or depressive episode.
Assess awareness of possible dangers to self of hypersexual behavior.	If unaware of danger to self from hypersexual acting-out behavior, additional protections may be needed, i.e., hospitalization.
Assess family/significant other's perception of changes in libido and consequences for family system.	Alteration in sexuality pattern of significant other can have marked effects on the dynamics of a family/couple system.
Provide interventions to maintain safety until changes in sexual behaviors are resolved.	Safety is maintained until acute phase of the illness is resolved.
Teach safe-sex practices.	Safety is maintained both during and after the acute phase of the illness.
Ineffective Individual Coping	
Assess ability to follow through with role(s) in life.	Illness may interfere with ability to care for self or others.
Ensure a safe physical and emotional environment until able to make reality-based decisions.	Depression and mania interfere with judgment and decision-making abilities. Helping with these processes will decrease frustration and maintain self-esteem.
Encourage continued problem-solving activities to allow for teaching and intervention.	The individual's sense of mastery over life is maintained and a forum for patient teaching is provided.
Present with reduced number of alternatives in decision making to minimize distraction/frustration.	This reduces need for selecting between choices and yet maintains feelings of independence and control over life.
Altered Thought Processes	
Assess ability to process instructions, follow conversations, and/or directions.	The severity of alteration in thought processes and ability to relate to others are determined.

Nursing Interventions	Rationales
Communicate in short, simple sentences.	This decreases complexity of communication in light of disorganized thought and allows for follow-through on conversation.
Redirect focus on topic of conversation	This allows for orientation to discussion and improves socialization skills.
Encourage consistency in daily schedule.	Consistent routines promote active participation in controlling daily life.

Altered Nutrition

Assess dietary intake and ongoing height/weight.	Mania and depression cause changes in appetite.
Encourage frequent snacks and adequate fluid intake if activity level interferes with meal time.	Manic patients have difficulty attending to tasks; thus, ensuring adequate food and fluid intake may necessitate creative interventions.
Encourage intake of nutritious, low-calorie foods if food intake is increased.	Depressed patients may overeat and underexercise, resulting in weight gain.
Limit the amount of caffeinated beverages in diet.	Caffeine stimulates the autonomic nervous system and increases levels of agitation.

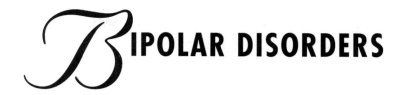

IPOLAR DISORDERS

Karen G. Vincent, MS, RN, CS

The term *Bipolar Disorder* refers to the extremes of the mood cycle: the hyperactivity and increased energy level experienced by patients with "mania" and the depressive end of the spectrum, with loss of motivation and energy and, sometimes, the total loss of goal-directed activity. Individuals with manic-depressive illness (Bipolar Disorder) experience swings between these extreme poles of mood in separate blocks of time. The individual episodes may last for weeks to months. Usually, when a client has recovered from a manic episode, it is common to witness a brief "reactive" depression before a return to baseline behavior and daily functioning. Manic-depressive illness afflicts equal numbers of men and women. The average age of onset of the illness is the early twenties.

The newest classification of Bipolar Disorders identifies two specific types: Bipolar I and II Disorders. The first term refers to those clients who present with a classic manic-depressive illness, i.e., fluctuations between manic highs and depressive lows with periods of remission in regular patterns. Bipolar II Disorder is manifested by recurrent episodes of Major Depression with documentation of hypomanic episodes experienced between the depressions. The treatments of these two types of illnesses are different and will be discussed in this chapter.

Clinical Clip

Cyclothymia, a subtype of manic-depressive illness, is experienced as a continuous fluctuation in mood between hypomania and depression. The episodes may last days to weeks (instead of months), but the periods between episodes are short-lived. The severity of the symptoms is, however, less than the bipolar disorders.

ETIOLOGIES
- Alteration in circadian rhythm
  - delayed sleep phase insomnia
  - malfunctioning of interpretation of environmental cues for sleep, e.g., light/darkness
  - reduced intensity or loss of circadian rhythm
- Catecholamine hypothesis: excess amount of neurotransmitters at postsynaptic site (of neurons in brain) during mania and depletion during depression
- Depletion of the neurotransmitter gamma-aminobutyric acid (GABA), which inhibits rapid firing of neurons in brain
- Abnormal amounts of neurotransmitters serotonin, dopamine, norepinephrine, and adrenocorticotropic hormone (ACTH)
- Thyroid levels: hypothyroidism
- Alteration in following endocrinology axes: hypothalamic-pituitary-adrenal and hypothalamic-pituitary-thyroid systems
- Establishment of genetic "markers" for Bipolar Disorder. Results of the Amish Study found genetic marker on chromosome 11 that increases an individual's vulnerability to develop the disorder (Kavanagh, 1991).

CLINICAL MANIFESTATIONS

Manic Episode Features
- Continuously elevated energy level
- Irritable and/or grandiose mood
- Easily distractible
- Racing thoughts
- Decreased need for sleep
- Feelings of infallibility, grandiosity, and no regard for consequences of behavior
- Poor judgment, i.e., spending sprees, hypersexuality
- Pressured speech
- Increased work pace, goal-directed activity
- Symptoms interfere with occupational and/or social functioning
- Not caused by abuse of substances

Depressive Episode Features
- Duration of symptoms for at least 2 weeks
- Depressed mood
- Anhedonia (loss of interest or pleasure in previously enjoyed activities)
- Fatigue
- Weight loss or gain
- Insomnia or hypersomnia
- Psychomotor agitation or retardation (slowed movements)
- Feelings of worthlessness and guilt
- Poor concentration
- Recurrent thoughts of death or suicide

CLINICAL/DIAGNOSTIC FINDINGS

- Positive family history of manic-depressive illness in a first-generation relative
- Mini–Mental Status Exam
  - inability to attend to questions
  - increased irritability
  - perseveration on content of questions
- Bipolar depression
  - Beck's Depression Inventory, score over 11
  - Zung's Self-Administered Depression Scale, score over 55
  - Hamilton's Rating Scale for Depression, score over 13

▶ NURSING DIAGNOSIS: *High Risk for Injury*

Risk Factors

- Impaired judgment (hypersexual acting-out behavior, grandiosity with no regard for consequences of behavior)
- Inability to sleep/sleep disturbance
- Irritability
- Poor concentration
- Suicidal ideation

Patient Outcomes

Patient will
- be free of injury during acute phase of illness.
- recognize behaviors that place them in potentially dangerous situations.

Nursing Interventions	Rationales
Assess judgment regarding activities that may be potentially dangerous.	Poor judgment and decision-making skills (secondary to mania and depression) place them at high risk for injury.
Assess attention span, ability to concentrate, and feelings of grandiosity and immortality.	Risk taking, hypersexuality, and decreased ability to concentrate due to racing thoughts are all risk factors for injury. Hospitalization may be required during the manic phase if the patient is unable to maintain safety.
Assess for suicidal ideation.	Depression often precipitates suicidal ideation.

Nursing Interventions	Rationales
Provide safe and structured environment, if necessary, to prevent injury during acute phase of illness.	Cognitive functions may be so impaired that hospitalization is necessary to protect the client. Interventions would need to be simple and concrete due to decreased attention span and poor reality testing about self-protective abilities.
Speak in short, simple sentences and make verbal limit setting concrete goals with few options.	Provide few options to prevent overwhelming decision-making processes while allowing as much independent control as possible.
Teach about high-risk behaviors that may be potentially harmful to self after the acute phase of the illness is over.	Ongoing therapy and/or intervention after the acute phase of the illness will assist with life-style management with a chronic illness that alters judgment.
Continually evaluate behaviors and response to environmental stimuli that may be harmful in the inpatient setting and community.	Assessment and reassessment with the client as partner are part of helping to deal with a life-long illness.

▶ **NURSING DIAGNOSIS:** *Impaired Social Interaction*

Related To symptoms of manic phase of illness, i.e., grandiosity, intrusive behavior, and pressured speech.

Defining Characteristics
- Observed use of unsuccessful social interaction behaviors
- Dysfunctional interaction with peers, family, and health care providers
- Observed inability to receive or communicate a sense of belonging, caring, or interest in others

Patient Outcomes
Patient will interact with others in a socially appropriate manner.

Nursing Interventions	Rationales
Assess quality of social interaction with family, peers, and health care providers.	Baseline data of behaviors are established that may be interfering with relationships.
Note reaction of others to interaction with patient	Material to use for feedback with client is provided regarding impact of behavior with others.
Assess insight into appropriateness of social interactions.	Poor judgment and manic behavior can cloud insight about impact of behavior on others.
Provide safe environment where patient will not be embarrassed by behavior upon recovery.	It may be necessary to limit social interactions with others on the unit when manic for several reasons: 1. Other patients may begin to get angry with manic patient. 2. A high degree of uncontrolled energy from one patient may escalate behavior on the entire unit. 3. The patient may experience extreme embarrassment about behavior once the manic episode is resolved.
Redirect to activities with minimal socialization.	A less stimulating environment is provided.
Set limits on behaviors that interfere with the therapeutic milieu.	Escalation of other patients' disorganized and potentially aggressive behaviors is prevented.
Evaluate feelings about manic episode and social behavior during the recovery phase.	Ventilation of feelings of remorse and/or embarrassment about behavior that may interfere with return to prior level of social functioning is allowed.

▶ NURSING DIAGNOSIS: *Noncompliance*

Related To
- Feelings of increased energy, elation, grandiosity, and infallibility
- Denial of need for medication
- Increased irritability

Defining Characteristics
- Behavior indicative of failure to adhere to medical regimen
  - refusing medication
  - "cheeking" medication and then disposing of it
- Decreased lithium levels
- Verbalization of lack of need for medications
- Evidence of exacerbation of symptoms
- Failure to keep appointments

Patient Outcomes
Patient will
- begin to comply with the therapeutic regimen.
- verbalize need to take medications.
- design own plan of care for after discharge with the health care team.

Nursing Interventions	Rationales
Assess history of noncompliance with health care regimen.	Baseline of frequency and consequences of not following through with medication and/or appointments are established.
Assess insight into need for medication to control symptoms of Bipolar Disorder.	This provides information about acceptance and knowledge about disorder as well as whether "manic highs" are perceived as enjoyable and productive states.
Involve family/significant others in education/follow-through with health care.	If family is involved in patient's life, illness will also affect them. Providing education and support will limit their feelings of burnout and enhance their ability to lend support.
Tailor the medication time schedule to life-style.	Feelings of control over the health care regimen are encouraged and follow-through with medication enhanced.
Reality test the pros and cons of manic highs vs. stable mood.	Often periods of manic behavior offer increased amounts of energy and productivity. Education must involve looking at the negative impact of manic episodes on personal life.

Nursing Interventions	Rationales
Evaluate follow-through and knowledge of purpose of medication and consistency with appointments after discharge.	The effectiveness of the interventions during admission is assessed. Continued care is more easily planned.

▶ NURSING DIAGNOSIS: *Ineffective Denial*

Related To
- Feelings of grandiosity
- Inability to accept chronic illness

Defining Characteristics
- Delays seeking health care attention to detriment of health
- Does not perceive personal relevance of symptoms or danger
- Minimizes symptoms
- Unable to admit impact of disorder on life style
- Makes dismissive gestures or comments when speaking of distressing events
- Displays inappropriate affect

Patient Outcomes
Patient will
- voluntarily seek help from mental health professsionals for exacerbation of symptoms.
- demonstrate acceptance of illness by actively participating in treatment process.

Nursing Interventions	Rationales
Assess knowledge about illness and its treatment.	Establishes learning needs vs. denial of severity of illness.
Explore past experiences with treatment and ability to engage with mental health team.	Provides background information regarding difficulty or ease of participating in therapy.
Assess present status of thought processes and judgment.	Current alterations in thought processes may contribute to denial and have an impact on treatment.
Reinforce need to follow through with treatment as a source of self-control.	Extends sense of mastery and control over illness to patient.

Nursing Interventions	Rationales
Engage family/significant others in treatment process.	Support from family system will encourage follow-through.
Evaluate ability to follow through with treatment over time.	Ability to follow through with treatment may change with mood cycles; information gained over time is important for future planning.

▶ NURSING DIAGNOSIS: *High Risk for Caregiver Role Strain*

Risk Factors
* Illness severity of care receiver
* Repeated cycle of illness with recurring hospitalizations
* Threats of violence to self and/or others in family
* Caregiver's coping patterns
* Caregiver exhibits bizarre behavior
* Past history of poor relationship with care receiver

Patient System Outcomes
Patient's caregivers will
* acknowledge stress involved in caring for family members.
* seek out support systems to deal with ongoing caregiving task.
Patient will
* exhibit absence of any signs of abuse/neglect in the home.

Nursing Interventions	Rationales
Assess caregiver's ability to care for the family member physically, emotionally, and financially.	Physical limitations of the caregiver, environmental barriers within the home, financial stressors, and additional caretaking responsibilities can all impact on the caregiver's ability to sustain the constant stress of caring for a person with mental/physical impairment.
Assess level of severity of cognitive impairment/functional status of patient.	Baseline data of functional cognitive limitations of patient and extent of caregiving tasks of family are established.

Nursing Interventions	Rationales
Note any disturbances in family system prior to onset of illness, i.e., alcohol/drug abuse, violence, and/or divorce.	Previously fragile family dynamics will be further stressed by a prolonged illness, and early intervention may prevent abuse or neglect.
Assess caregiver's coping strategies.	Maladaptive coping strategies can lead to burnout, anger with the affected family member, and potential abuse. Resources to help refocus the caregiver's coping abilities will assist the family unit.
Ask whether there have been episodes of striking out/violent acts toward family members.	Interventions with medications may be necessary to ensure the safety of the family members. Also, family may be helped to incorporate behavioral techniques into the care of their loved one.
Evaluate family's understanding of illness.	Coping skills are compromised when there is uncertainty. Misinformation or an incorrect perception of an illness, i.e., diagnosis, treatment, and expected progression can limit the family's ability to prepare for the care.
Teach family about illness, i.e., course and progression.	Education is known to alleviate anxiety surrounding illness. It helps the family/patient feel more in control of the disease and anticipating care needs.
Encourage family/caregiver to seek external support for help.	Social support systems outside of the family will provide emotional outlets, validation of feelings/grief about family member's illness, and ability to express feelings about the stigma of mental illness.
Evaluate status of ongoing caregiving during progression of patient's illness. Be ready to act as an advocate and support system for the family, whether patient is in the hospital, a nursing home, or at home.	Involving the family in the care planning and care will provide needed social support.

CONTINUITY OF CARE/DISHARGE PLANNING

- Individual therapy to provide support, follow symptoms, and monitor medication blood levels
- Inpatient hospitalization if needed for dangerous behavior toward self or others
- Refer for group and/or family therapy
- Refer to community-based support groups and to National Depressive and Manic-Depressive Association, 730 North Franklin St., Suite 501, Chicago, IL 60610, 1-800/82-NDMDA

BIBLIOGRAPHY

American Psychiatric Association (APA). (1994). *Diagnostic and statistical manual of mental disorders* (4th ed.). Washington, DC: APA.

Cook, S. & Fontaine, K. (1991). *Essentials of mental health nursing,* 2nd Edition. Redwood City, CA: Addison-Wesley.

Kavanaugh, C. (1991). Psychiatric-mental health nursing: The nursing process. In F. Gary & C. Kavanaugh (Ed.) *Psychiatric-mental health nursing,* pp. 12–13. Philadelphia, PA: Lippincott.

North American Nursing Diagnosis Association (1992). *NANDA nursing diagnosis: definitions and classification 1992–1993.* St. Louis, MO: NANDA.

Oaykel, E. S. (Ed.) (1992). *Handbook of affective disorders,* 2nd Edition. New York: Guilford Press.

United States Department of Health and Human Services (USDHHS). Public Health Service, Agency for Health Care Policy and Research (AHCPR). (1993). *Depression in primary care: Clinical practice guidelines number 5.* Publication No. 93-0550. Rockville, MD: USDHHS.

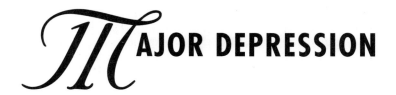

AJOR DEPRESSION

Karen G. Vincent, MS, RN, CS

Major Depression is the most common type of affective disorder, afflicting one in eight individuals in the United States (4.4 per 100 individuals in the Epidemiological Catchment Area Study done in the 1980s). It is a debilitating disorder which impacts all spheres of a persons life: social, occupational, physical, and emotional. Women are affected by major depression in larger numbers than men. Major Depression is labeled "unipolar" because the individual does not experience episodes of mania, in addition to the depressive symptoms.

Clinical Clip

Dysthmic Disorder is a subtype of depression characterized by persistent but not debilitating symptoms of depression that exist for more than two years.

ETIOLOGIES
- Genetic transmission: first-degree relatives with bipolar or unipolar disorders or substance abuse
- Deficiency of neurotransmitter amine at postsynaptic neuronal site; neurotransmitters include dopamine, norepinephrine, and serotonin
- Excess of monoamine oxidase, which depletes neurotransmitters in brain
- Reduced sensitivity of neuronal receptor sites themselves
- Alteration in limbic system area of brain, which controls affective states such as pleasure, mood, and activity levels
- Hypersensitivity to environmental stressors, which then affects the neurotransmitter centers of the brain
- Circadian rhythms: biochemical (melatonin) response to changes in light during winter (seasonal affective disorder)
- Complicated or unresolved bereavement

- External locus of control theories (e.g., depending on others for self-esteem)
- Learned helplessness: psychological sequela is depression
- Cognitive theory includes three components: negative views of self, present and future; negative ways of interpreting environmental stimuli; and cognitive or judgmental errors in thinking
- Medical illnesses
- Side effects from medication or polypharmacy

CLINICAL MANIFESTATIONS
- Duration of symptoms for at least 2 weeks
- Depressed mood
- Anhedonia (loss of interest or pleasure in previously enjoyed activities)
- Fatigue
- Weight loss or gain
- Insomnia or hypersomnia
- Psychomotor agitation or retardation (slowed movements)
- Feelings of worthlessness and guilt
- Poor concentration
- Recurrent thoughts of death or suicide

CLINICAL/DIAGNOSTIC FINDINGS
- Complete physical examination which would ascertain any underlying or undiagnosed medical illness that can mimic depression, e.g.,
  - Parkinson's disease
  - hyper- /hypothyroidism
  - diabetes
  - carcinoma
  - pneumonia
  - acquired immunodeficiency syndrome (AIDS)
- Clean catch urine to rule out urinary tract infections or underlying infections, which also mimic depression, especially in elderly
- Chest x-ray to rule out pneumonia or lesions
- Complete review of current medications to
  - determine polypharmacy reactions
  - establish whether some medications (such as digoxin, propranalol, indomethacin) are causing secondary depression
- Beck's Depression Inventory (score over 11)
- Zung Self-Rating Depression Scale (score over 55)
- Hamilton Rating Scale for Depression (score over 13)

▶ NURSING DIAGNOSIS: *High Risk for Violence—Directed at Self*

Risk Factors
- Prior history of suicidal gestures/attempts
- Drug/alcohol abuse
- Family history of suicide
- Increasing anxiety levels
- Advanced age

- Presence of depression
- Available means
- Verbalized intent/plans for suicide

- Physical illnesses
- Presence of psychotic symptoms
- Lack of social supports

Patient Outcomes

Patient will

- verbalize ideas of suicidal intent with health care providers.
- contract for safety and plans to contact significant others or health care providers if ideation of danger to self increases.
- begin to make plans for the future after the acute phase of the depression.

Nursing Interventions	Rationales
Assess for presence of risk factors for suicide, such as age, past history of suicide attempts, and/or substance abuse.	Risk factors have been documented to increase the potential for self-harm.
Assess whether patient has plans and viable means to carry out the attempt.	A thorough suicide plan and the means to carry it out increase the danger of success.
Assess status of social supports.	Social supports are an essential component of helping the depressed client through the worst part of the illness.
Discuss safety contract.	Alliance with health care team is built if patient can contract for safety.
Use empathetic listening and communication techniques.	Conveys genuine caring and concern when the person cannot care for self.
Evaluate for potential of self-harm and hospitalize if necessary.	Hospitalization may be necessary if patient is acutely suicidal and cannot contract for safety.
Remove any dangerous article from area and assign staff to sit with patient.	This conveys sense of caring for safety and being attentive to needs, so patient does not have to act out to ask for help.
Reassure that feelings of hopelessness and despair remit with antidepressant medication.	A sense of hope is provided based on realistic treatment issues.

Nursing Interventions	Rationales
Evaluate suicidal potential on an ongoing basis until 14–21 days after medication has been initiated.	Patients are most at risk when energy level begins to respond to antidepressant medication and yet mood has not altered.

▶ NURSING DIAGNOSIS: *Social Isolation*

Related To preoccupation with internal life and other vegetative symptoms of depression.

Defining Characteristics
- Sad, dull affect
- Uncommunicative
- Withdrawn
- No eye contact
- Preoccupation with own thoughts
- Seeks to be alone
- Experiences feelings of difference from others
- Absence of significant purpose in life

Patient Outcomes
Patient will
- attend groups and meals on unit as assigned.
- begin to interact with peers and staff on unit.
- increase social interactions with family and friends.

Nursing Interventions	Rationales
Assess level of interaction with peers and staff on unit.	Baseline interaction on unit is determined and a guide for judging improvement provided.
Ask family/significant other about past socialization patterns.	Past level of socialization is formulated so that interventions and outcomes can be monitored.
Encourage to attend unit performance groups and meal times.	Expectations of and self-mastery over symptoms are set.
Help to minimize the number of negative self-verbalizations in groups.	Personal interactions within groups are normalized.
Evaluate social interaction via behavior on unit and input from family system.	The success of milieu interventions and medication response are ascertained.

▶ NURSING DIAGNOSIS: *Self-Esteem Disturbance*

Related To
- Learned helplessness
- Exaggerated and often unfounded feelings of shame/guilt resulting from biochemical imbalances in brain

Defining Characteristics
- Self-negating verbalizations
- Expressions of shame/guilt
- Evaluating self as unable to deal with events
- Exaggerating negative feedback about self
- Hypersensitive to slight or criticism

Patient Outcomes
Patient will
- decrease the number of self-negating comments.
- identify strengths and abilities.
- verbalize positive self-concept.

Nursing Interventions	Rationales
Assess negative thought patterns for logic, validity, and frequency; reality test with client.	Depressed clients tend to ruminate on negative issues, especially self-worth.
Assist to set realistic expectations for self.	Realistic expectations help to reality test about self-negating thoughts and provide goal setting and structure in treatment.
Encourage to attend groups or unit activities to break the pattern of self-criticism.	Attention directed outside of self will result in diminished intrusive thoughts.
Teach that negative ruminations about the self are a part of depression and treatable with medications.	Education can provide relief that thoughts are related to the depression and enables patient to feel control over monitoring progress.
Assess whether repeating thought patterns have been present before in patient's life.	This provides information about existence of negative self-constructs in thinking before the onset of depression.
Evaluate frequency of occurrence of negative thoughts as treatment progresses.	Such evaluations allow for assessment of success of milieu and medical treatment.

▶ NURSING DIAGNOSIS: *Hopelessness*

Related To
- Inability to choose between alternatives
- Perceiving few or no choices available
- Lethargy as ongoing vegetative symptom of depression

Defining Characteristics
- Passivity
- Decreased verbalizations
- Decreased eye contact
- Increased sighing
- Lack of initiative
- Shrugging in response to speaker
- Decreased appetite

Patient Outcomes
Patient will
- begin to participate in unit activities.
- verbalize positive expectations for the future.

Nursing Interventions	Rationales
Assess level of hopelessness via plans/expectations for the future.	Hopelessness results in tunnel vision about the promise of the future.
Assess past coping skills.	Past coping skills may be overwhelmed by present stressors in life.
Provide an open, therapeutic relationship.	The patient can begin to trust and verbalize feelings related to hopelessness.
Assure patient that hopelessness is a symptom of depression.	Feelings are verified and a viable framework that feelings will improve is provided.
Encourage participation in unit groups and activities.	Stimulation and opportunities to express emotions are provided.
Encourage family/significant others to visit.	This breaks the self-imposed isolation created by hopeless feelings.

▶ NURSING DIAGNOSIS: *Powerlessness*

Related To lack of intrapsychic energy to make decisions and actively participate in life.

Defining Characteristics
- Verbal expression of having no control or influence over situation or outcome
- Nonparticipation in decision making
- Expression of doubt regarding role performance
- Passivity
- Inability to seek information regarding care
- Dependence on others that may result in irritability, resentment, anger, and guilt

Patient Outcomes
Patient will demonstrate active involvement in life's activities.

Nursing Interventions	Rationales
Assess for impact of feelings of powerlessness on life and relationships with others.	Severity of feelings of powerlessness is determined.
Assess prior incidents of feelings of powerlessness.	Whether this behavior is new or a repeating pattern is established.
Establish a therapeutic relationship.	A forum is provided for reviewing past relationship styles and practicing new ways of relating.
Discuss feelings about making needs known, and fears about expressing self.	Results of being assertive, past experiences with same, and feelings about making new attempts to be assertive are verified.
Help to set realistic daily goals over which patient has control.	A sense of mastery and a sense of self control are established.

CONTINUITY OF CARE/DISCHARGE PLANNING
- Initiate individual therapy to provide support, follow symptoms, and monitor medication blood levels.
- Inpatient hospitalization as needed for exacerbation of symptoms.
- Refer for group and/or family therapy.

- Refer to community-based support groups and to the National Depressive and Manic Depressive Association, 730 North Franklin St., Suite 501, Chicago, IL 60610.

BIBLIOGRAPHY

Burgess, A. (1990). *Psychiatric nursing in the hospital and the community* (5th ed.). Norwalk, CT: Appleton & Lange.

Cook, S., & Fontaine, K. (1991). *Essentials of mental health nursing* (2nd ed.). Redwood City, CA: Addison-Wesley.

Gettrust, K., & Brabec, P. (1992). *Nursing diagnosis in clinical practice: Guides for care planning.* Albany, NY: Delmar.

Mondimore, F. (1993). *Depression: The mood disorder.* Baltimore, MD: Johns Hopkins University Press.

North American Nursing Diagnosis Association (NANDA). (1992). *NANDA nursing diagnoses: Definitions and classification 1992–1993.* St. Louis, MO: NANDA.

Paykel, E. S. (Ed.). (1992). *Handbook of affective disorders* (2nd ed.). New York: Guilford.

Task Force on *DSM-IV*, American Psychiatric Association (APA). (1993). *DSM-IV draft criteria.* Washington, DC: APA.

United States Department of Health and Human Services (USDHHS), Public Health Service, Agency for Health Care Policy and Research (AHCPR). (1993). *Depression in primary care: Clinical practice guideline number 5.* Publication No. 93-0550. Rockville, MD: USDHHS.

Anxiety Disorders

Joan Norris, PhD, RN

Anxiety Disorders are characterized by physical and psychological symptoms of anxiety and/or behaviors undertaken in order to avoid anxiety or related situations. The lifetime prevalence of these disorders is reported to be 14.6% in the United States, as reported by the Epidemiologic Catchment Area Study. At present, there is extensive exploration of familial, biochemical and behavioral factors in the development and treatment of these disorders (Schatzberg, 1991). The *Diagnostic and Statistical Manual of Mental Disorders 4th ed.* identifies the following disorders in this category:

- Panic Attack—a sudden intense fear/discomfort with defined cognitive or somatic symptoms (i.e., palpitations, trembling, nausea).
- Agoraphobia—anxiety of being in a situation or place from which escape is difficult or impossible.
- Panic Disorder—recurrent, unexpected panic attacks with persistent concern of having another; may be with or without Agoraphobia.
- Agoraphobia without History of Panic Disorder—similar to Panic Disorder with Agoraphobia, but fear is focused on incapacitating or embarrassing panic-type symptoms.
- Specific Phobia—fear of discernible objects or situations.
- Social Phobia—fear of social or performance situations that may cause embarrassment, provoke anxiety. The fear is recognized as excessive and unreasonable.
- Obsessive-Compulsive Disorder—distressing, recurring obsessions or compulsions that are time-consuming.

- Posttraumatic Stress Disorder—the reexperiencing of a traumatic event that causes increased arousal and trauma associated with stimulus avoidance.
- Acute Stress Disorder—symptoms similar to posttraumatic stress disorder occurring immediately after a traumatic event.
- Generalized Anxiety Disorder—excessive anxiety occurring more days than not for at least 6 months.
- Anxiety Disorder Due to a Medical Condition—judged to be due to the physiological effects of a medical condition.
- Substance-Induced Anxiety Disorder—judged to be due to the effects of a substance.

The nursing syndrome for anxiety is best represented by the human response patterns feeling, choosing, perceiving, knowing, and relating as follows:

HRP	Nursing Diagnosis	Related To
Feeling	Anxiety	Unknown, vague distress with sympathetic nervous system arousal
	Fear	Concern about exposure to specific objects (phobia) or inability to predict or control future anxiety attacks
	Posttrauma response	Prior exposure to violent or other distressing events beyond the normal range of experience
	Rape-trauma syndrome	Prior experience of forced sex activity by family member, peer, or stranger
Relating	Impaired social interaction	Avoidance/withdrawal from social activities
Perceiving	Self-esteem disturbance	Inability to control symptoms or behavior, powerlessness, shame, or embarrassment
	Powerlessness	Inability to control symptoms or behavior
Knowing	Altered thought processes	Panic levels of anxiety
Choosing	Ineffective management of therapeutic regimen	Hopelessness, lack of knowledge, depression
	Ineffective family coping	Disrupted family dynamics and relationships
	Family coping: potential for growth	Family interest in gaining knowledge, skills, and support to enhance coping

Nursing Interventions	Rationales
Initiate cognitive-behavioral therapy (exposure/desensitization, relaxation/biofeedback, restructuring cognitions).	Fear/avoidance with approach tendencies is countered and a sense of mastery/control over feelings and behavior is promoted.
Engage in supportive group therapy.	Feedback and reinforcement in a climate of hopefulness are provided:
Institute and monitor pharmacotherapy: 1. benzodiazepines 2. tricyclic antidepressants 3. monoamine oxidase inhibitor (MAOI) antidepressants	1. useful in reducing panic and anticipatory anxiety 2. control panic attacks and reduce compulsions and depression 3. effective in phobia and agoraphobia

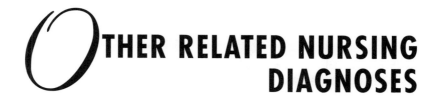

OTHER RELATED NURSING DIAGNOSES

Joan Norris, PhD, RN

▶ **NURSING DIAGNOSIS:** *Impaired Social Interaction*

Related To
- Avoidance of anxiety-provoking situations
- Excessive time devoted to ritualistic behavior
- Avoidance of interpersonal contact

Defining Characteristics
- Verbalized or observed discomfort in social situations
- Verbalized or observed inability to receive or communicate a satisfying sense of belonging, caring, interest, or shared history
- Unsuccessful social interaction behaviors
- Report of change of style and amount or pattern of interaction

Patient Outcomes
Patient will achieve (or reestablish) significant interpersonal-social relationships.

Nursing Interventions	Rationales
Observe social interactions and explore feelings about and barriers to satisfying interactions with patient.	Identification of the nature of the problem will assist with planning appropriate interventions.
Identify reasonable goals and activities for increasing/improving social interaction with the patient.	Mutual goal setting and planning promote goal attainment.

Nursing Interventions	Rationales
Acknowledge and reinforce patient for increased social activities and relationships.	Reinforcement increases likelihood that behavior will be repeated.
Teach value of social support to health and well-being.	Awareness of value of interaction can serve to motivate social efforts.

▶ NURSING DIAGNOSIS: *Powerlessness*

Related To perceived inability to predict and control anxiety-based thoughts, behavior, and feelings.

Defining Characteristics
- Verbal expressions of lacking control over situation
- Verbal expressions of having no control over self-care
- Verbal expressions of having no control/influence over outcomes
- Depression over deteriorating condition
- Does not monitor progress
- Expresses doubt about role performance
- Reluctant to express feelings or seek information

Patient Outcomes
Patient will experience increased feelings of hope, self-efficacy, and control.

Nursing Interventions	Rationales
Assess for feelings of powerlessness and depression.	Perceived powerlessness reduces active involvement in treatment and promotes depression.
Explore patient's reasons or experiences that underlie powerlessness and provide information about available choices and techniques to achieve greater control.	Appropriate exploration and education can increase hope and participation in treatment.
Carefully/gradually increase goals and skill training to maximize opportunities for success.	Excessive demands can result in failure and reinforce perceived powerlessness. Success experiences will promote and reinforce feelings of self-efficacy and control.
Teach cognitive restructuring to stop negative thoughts of	Negative self-talk reinforces powerlessness. Substituting positive

Nursing Interventions	Rationales
powerlessness and substitute reality-based thoughts of hope and control.	self-talk reinforces a sense of realistic ability to master problems.

▶ NURSING DIAGNOSIS: *Self-Esteem Disturbance (Chronic or Situational)*

Related To
- Negative self-evaluation of role performance or capabilities
- Perceived powerlessness or helplessness
- Changes in energy level or capabilities
- Loss of emotional or behavioral control

Defining Characteristics
- Verbalizes inability to deal with events
- Exaggerates negative feedback about self
- Expresses shame or guilt
- Indecisive
- Minimizes or rationalizes away positive feedback
- Verbalizes self-negating/derogatory statements

Patient Outcomes
Patient will increasingly
- recognize self as a person of value.
- identify assets and personal strengths.
- express feelings and needs appropriately.
- express feelings of personal competence.

Nursing Interventions	Rationales
Assess for duration and perceived factors associated with low self-esteem and for any associated depression or suicidal thoughts.	Identification of duration and depth of the problem and any associated problems are vital to planning care and promoting patient participation.
Initiate therapeutic relationship.	Acceptance and respect on the part of the nurse promote self-acceptance and growth.
Conduct a positive asset search.	Identifying assets serves to reinforce existing self-worth and identify strengths for treatment tasks.

Nursing Interventions	**Rationales**
Teach cognitive-behavioral skills of assertiveness and cognitive restructuring as needed.	Increased assertion is likely to result in reinforcing feelings of competence. If negative self-talk reinforces low self-esteem or feelings of inadequacy, patients can be taught to replace these negative thoughts with realistic assessments of strengths.

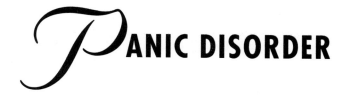

ᏙANIC DISORDER

Joan Norris, PhD, RN

Panic Attacks are episodes of fear and distress with at least four symptoms of sympathetic nervous system arousal, such as dyspnea, faintness, sweating, and rapid heart rate, not based on organic factors. Agoraphobia, anxiety about being in situations in which a panic attack may occur with no help or escape available, leads to avoidance of travel outside the home or enduring it despite great distress. Panic Disorders are then further classified as occurring without or with Agoraphobia and specifying the level of severity as mild, moderate, or severe. Distinguishing between Panic Disorder With Agoraphobia and the presence of Simple or Social Phobias may be difficult, particularly in persons who no longer experience Panic Attacks.

ETIOLOGIES
- Familial and biological factors
- Absence of organic factors such as hyperthyroidism, amphetamine use, and excessive caffeine intake
- Mitral valve prolapse may be associated
- Onset of symptoms most common in later twenties
- More common in women than in men

CLINICAL MANIFESTATIONS
- Frequent episodes (four in a month) with four or more of the following symptoms occurring during one or more of the attacks:
  - dyspnea or feelings of smothering/choking
  - vertigo, feelings of faintness or unsteadiness
  - rapid heart rate or palpitations
  - tremors, diaphoresis, and gastrointestinal (GI) upset
  - tingling sensations and/or feelings of unreality
  - hot flashes or chills
  - fears of dying or "going crazy"

CLINICAL/DIAGNOSTIC FINDINGS

- Panic Disorders are characterized by the absence of organic factors such as stimulant use or hyperthyroidism. Attacks may be induced in many already diagnosed individuals by sodium lactate injections or CO_2 inhalations.

▶ NURSING DIAGNOSIS: *Altered Thought Processes*

Related To severe to panic-level anxiety episodes.

Defining Characteristics

- Altered abstract thinking
- Distractibility, difficulty concentrating
- Indecisiveness
- Hypervigilance
- Inaccurate interpretation of stimuli
- Intrusive thoughts
- Memory problems

Patient Outcomes

Patient will develop
- awareness of own anxiety level and ability to identify signs/symptoms of acute anxiety.
- improved ability to interpret environmental stimuli and understand information.

Nursing Interventions	Rationales
Assess anxiety level and convey acceptance and observations.	Patient can recognize heightened anxiety without arousing defensiveness or embarrassment.
Modify communication.	Brief, clear sentences and evaluating patient's understanding of statements or questions serves to prevent any misinterpretation.
Reduce stimuli from environment as needed.	Simplifying the input from the environment reduces distractibility and distortion of information.
Reinforce key information and provide written instructions as needed.	Repetition and written instructions serve to compensate for distractibility and memory problems.
Offer reassurance that loss of concentration is temporary and due to anxiety.	The knowledge that concentration will improve serves to focus and motivate the patient to deal with underlying problems.

▶ NURSING DIAGNOSIS: *Anxiety*

Related To fear and distress.

Defining Characteristics
- Increased tension
- Apprehension
- Helplessness (painful and persistent)
- Uncertainty, increased wariness
- Fearful, scared, overexcited, jittery, shaky
- Distressed, worried, fear of nonspecific consequences
- Sympathetic stimulation [peripheral vasoconstriction, increased heart rate/blood pressure (BP), pupil dilation, perspiration]
- Expresses concerns

Patient Outcomes
Patient will increasingly
- recognize signs and symptoms of anxiety.
- master relaxation or biofeedback techniques.
- restructure negative thoughts to create a positive attitude for learning control of feelings and behavior.

Nursing Interventions	Rationales
Complete a history, physical, and substance use assessment.	These procedures rule out organic factors and identify the degree of interference with functioning and identify coexisting problems of depression or substance abuse related to anxiety.
Teach patient about dealing with anxiety.	Information about the nature of anxiety and the symptoms can remove fear of dying and form a basis for understanding treatment.
Practice and role play behavioral techniques.	These provide feedback and reinforcement for coping through positive anxiety management strategies, such as relaxation, biofeedback.
Teach skills of cognitive restructuring.	Reinterpreting/reducing threatening cues fosters sense of mastery/control.

Nursing Interventions	Rationales
Teach and monitor prescribed medication use and withdrawal (antianxiety and antidepressant drugs). Avoid use of nonprescription drugs and alcohol.	Abrupt discontinuation of medication may lead to dependency and withdrawal symptoms.
Promote confrontation of feared situations, not avoidance.	Agoraphobia can severely limit functioning; patients need support to cope and overcome avoidance.

DISCHARGE PLANNING/CONTINUITY OF CARE
- Initiate education and behavioral therapy since these are generally effective in the outpatient treatment of panic disorder.
- Encourage intensive brief therapy, which provides the behavioral skills for anxiety management behavior.
- Institute imipramine and exposure treatment, which lead to long-term improvement on general measures of panic, avoidance, and depression.
- Educate family members to promote understanding of the nature of the condition and symptoms and how to be appropriately supportive to the patient.

BIBLIOGRAPHY
American Psychiatric Association (APA). (1994). *Diagnostic and statistical manual of mental disorders* (4th ed.). Washington, DC: APA.

North American Nursing Diagnosis Association (NANDA). (1992). *NANDA nursing diagnoses: Definitions and classification*. St. Louis, MO: NANDA.

Schatzberg, A. (1991). Overview of anxiety disorders: Prevalence, biology, course and treatment. *Journal of Clinical Psychiatry, 52*(7), 5–9.

Task Force on *DSM-IV*, American Psychiatric Association (APA). (1991). *DSM-IV options book: Work in progress*. Washington, DC: APA.

Zinbarg, R., Barlow, D., Brown, T., & Hertz, R. (1992). Cognitive-behavioral approaches to the nature and treatment of anxiety disorders. *Annual Review of Psychology, 43*, 235–267.

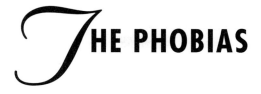

THE PHOBIAS

Joan Norris, PhD, RN

SOCIAL PHOBIA

Social Phobia is a persistent fear of being in situations in which one is likely to do something to cause embarrassment or ridicule, such as trembling or choking when speaking or eating in public. Exposure to the feared object or situation causes acute symptoms of anxiety, similar to panic, despite the individual's recognition that the fear is irrational. Avoidance of these situations is common. If a general medical condition, substance ingestion, and/or a mental disorder that cause severe embarrassment exist concurrently, the diagnosis of Social Phobia is not appropriate.

SPECIFIC (SIMPLE) PHOBIA

Specific (Simple) Phobia is a persistent fear of a specific object or situation such as enclosed spaces (claustrophobia), flying, animals, or heights. Confrontation with the feared stimulus causes severe anxiety which decreases as distance from the feared object increases.

ETIOLOGIES
- Unknown.
- Phobic clients may selectively attend to more threatening stimuli.
- Social Phobias may be reinforced by a vicious cycle of anticipatory anxiety that interferes with performance and further reinforces future anxiety.
- Onset most commonly in adolescence or young adulthood.
- Simple Phobias more common in females; Social Phobias may be slightly more common in females but males more frequently found in clinical populations.
Panic Disorder and Social and Simple (specific) Phobias may coexist.

CLINICAL MANIFESTATIONS
- The feared object or situation
  - evokes severe anxiety on exposure.
  - is avoided or tolerated only with great distress.
  - is recognized as unreasonable (APA, 1994).

CLINICAL/DIAGNOSTIC FINDINGS
- Increased heart rate, respirations, blood pressure (BP)
- Pallor
- Diaphoresis

▶ NURSING DIAGNOSIS: *Fear*

Related To an intense, unreasonable anticipation of a specific situation or object.

Defining Characteristics
- Feeling of dread
- Able to define specific object of fear
- Apprehensive, frightened, scared, afraid
- Terrified, panicky, jittery
- Increased tension, alarm, impulsiveness
- Decreased self-assurance
- Physiological signs: increased heart rate, respirations, and BP; gastrointestinal symptoms; pallor; diaphoresis; dilated pupils
- Withdrawal or aggression

Patient Outcomes
Patient will increasingly
- practice/master techniques of relaxation.
- practice/master exposure to the feared stimulus.
- substitute approach for avoidance behaviors.

Nursing Interventions	Rationales
Assess degree of interference with normal functioning, presence of depression, and substance use.	Depression and substance abuse may coexist. Monitor functioning to assess improvement.
Teach techniques of relaxation and process of desensitization.	Understanding and participation of client is elicited.
Practice confrontation with stimulus in conditions of relaxation; monitor and reinforce client progress.	Reinforcers promote hope and behavior change, as does the increased sense of behavior control.

CONTINUITY OF CARE/DISCHARGE PLANNING

- Initiate brief, behavioral exposure therapy. (A single 2-hr session has been effective in some cases.)
- Teach cognitive restructuring which reduces the tendency to distort cues and catastrophize events.
- Prescribe monoamine oxidase inhibitors as needed. (The presence of depression or substance abuse, if untreated, may interfere with improvement.)

BIBLIOGRAPHY

American Psychiatric Association (APA) (1994). *Diagnostic and statistical manual of mental disorders.* (4th ed.). Washington, DC: APA.

North American Nursing Diagnosis Association (NANDA). (1992). *Definitions and classification.* St. Louis, MO: NANDA.

Task Force on *DSM-IV,* American Psychiatric Association (APA). (1991). *DSM-IV options book: Work in progress.* Washington, DC: APA.

Whitley, G. (1992). Concept analysis of fear. *Nursing Diagnosis, 3*(2), 155–161.

Zinbarg, R., Barlow, D., Brown, T., & Hertz, R. (1992). Cognitive-behavioral approaches to the nature and treatment of anxiety disorders. *Annual Review of Psychology, 43,* 235–267.

OBSESSIVE-COMPULSIVE DISORDER

Joan Norris, PhD, RN

Obsessions are recurrent thoughts, visual images, or urges that cause severe anxiety. Clients strive to rid themselves of these thoughts or neutralize them through repetitious acts and are aware that the thoughts originate in their own minds. Common obsessions include violent impulses, becoming infected through contact with objects or people, and concerns that one has caused an injury. Compulsions are recurrent, ritualistic behaviors that are designed to relieve the distress caused by obsessions. Common compulsions include washing, rechecking, and counting activities. The person is aware that these behaviors are excessive, ritualistic, and not reasonable. Tension and anxiety increase with attempts to resist performing rituals; relief occurs following the compulsive behavior. Normal functioning is impaired because inordinate amounts of time are required for the obsessive thinking and compulsive behavior, which takes away from work, family, and social role activities.

ETIOLOGIES
- Not known
- Familial and biological factors (possibly)
- Adolescent or early adult onset common
- Men and women fairly equally represented

CLINICAL MANIFESTATIONS
- Obsessions and/or compulsions cause serious distress and take up more than 1 hr per day or interfere with functioning.
- Depression and substance abuse may be complications of the Obsessive-Compulsive Disorder (OCD).

CLINICAL/DIAGNOSTIC FINDINGS

- Brain imaging may reveal abnormalities of the frontal lobe and basal ganglia.

▶ NURSING DIAGNOSIS: *Anxiety*

Related To persistent, ego-dystonic thoughts.

Defining Characteristics

- Increased tension
- Apprehension
- Distress
- Fear of nonspecific consequences
- Sympathetic stimulation: [increased heart rate, respiration, blood pressure (BP); diaphoresis; dilated pupils; peripheral vasoconstriction]
- Expressed concerns

Patient Outcomes

Patient will increasingly
- reduce time in performing rituals.
- learn to delay rituals to an appropriate time.
- substitute positive anxiety management practices.
- learn to express thoughts and feelings.
- schedule time to include normal and recreational activities.

Nursing Interventions	Rationales
Assess anxiety level, health status, and degree of interference with normal activities/roles.	Identifying physical problems and life-style interferences helps determine priorities for care.
Direct patient to record the duration and context of rituals.	Recording duration and context of rituals helps in the planning for length of gradual exposure to situations that trigger ritualistic behaviors.
Teach and practice inhibiting/delaying rituals, substituting activities such as physical exercise to reduce anxiety.	Prevention of anxiety escalation reduces tension and interrupts pattern of ritualistic behavior.
If used, teach patient about clomipramine therapy and monitor therapy.	Clomipramine reduces the urgency of obsessions and compulsions. Knowledge of use and side effects reduces uncertainty about therapy.

Nursing Interventions	Rationales
Encourage expression of thoughts and feelings.	Opportunities for safe expression in a climate of acceptance promotes open communication.
Teach and assist to schedule times for normal activities, anxiety management, and leisure.	Enlisting patient in planning and problem solving promotes adherence to therapeutic plan.

▶ NURSING DIAGNOSIS: *Ineffective Management of Therapeutic Regimen*

Related To
- Complexity of therapeutic tasks
- Decisional conflicts
- Inadequate number and types of cues to action
- Minimizing perceived seriousness
- Powerlessness
- Lack of adequate social support

Defining Characteristics
- Choices of daily living ineffective for meeting goals of treatment program
- Verbalized desire to manage treatment
- Verbalized difficulty with integration of one or more prescribed treatments/actions
- Verbalization that desired action to reduce risk of progression or sequelae was not taken

Patient Outcomes
Patient will
- verbalize understanding of all necessary components of the treatment regimen.
- participate in planning and evaluating the integration of the prescribed treatment/activities into daily activities.

Nursing Interventions	Rationales
Educate patient as to the nature of the disorder and the relationship of the therapeutic regimen to attainment of mutually derived goals.	The patient's understanding and participation are vital to motivating effort and commitment to regimen.

Nursing Interventions	Rationales
Evaluate patient's understanding of all necessary tasks/activities.	
Assess readiness to undertake regimen activities.	Assessment of readiness is essential for identifying the current level of motivation to adapt to and participate in care.
Involve patient in planning and problem solving the integration of regimen activities into daily life.	Individualization of the regimen and removal of barriers to implementation are necessary to integration process.
Select and implement strategies to promote change as needed: 1. Promote self-confrontation (assist patient to recognize the problem and experience dissatisfaction with current behavior or lifestyle). 2. Teach cognitive restructuring to modify self-defeating beliefs and negative self-talk. 3. Provide modeling to demonstrate specific behaviors associated with positive changes. 4. Teach self-modification skills (self-assessment, reinforcement, and monitoring of target behaviors).	1. Assisting the person to acknowledge deficits/discrepancies between valued goals and current behavior can stimulate awareness of need for change. 2. Changing negative self-statements and beliefs/expectations permits positive ideation and behaviors to emerge and be reinforced. 3. Selection of appropriate models or demonstration of key behaviors permits covert (internal) rehearsal of positive behaviors. 4. Providing behavioral management skills permits sense of self-control and mastery.

▶ NURSING DIAGNOSIS: *Ineffective Family Coping (Compromised) or Family Coping (Potential for Growth)*

Related To disruption of family functions (and/or) relationships caused by preoccupation with obsessions and ritualistic activities.

Defining Characteristics

Compromised
- Family expresses concern about patient problem.
- Family expresses concern about members' reactions to patient problem.
- Significant person expresses inadequate understanding.
- Significant person withdraws or displays disproportionate protective behavior.

Potential for Growth
- Family supports growth and maturation of members.
- Family monitors treatment and makes choices promoting wellness.
- Family expresses interest in meeting with others who have experienced similar situations for mutual support.

Family/Significant Other Outcomes
Family/significant other will
- understand the disorder and its treatment.
- distinguish between supportive and nonsupportive behaviors for the OCD patient and family.
- identify support persons or groups in the community.

Nursing Interventions	Rationales
Educate family or significant other about the condition and its treatment.	Knowledge of the condition assists in relieving uncertainty and feelings of shame or blame.
Discuss with patient and family those actions which will be growth-supporting.	Participation of all will open communication and identify approaches that are helpful and promote clarity and consistency.
Review available support persons and groups.	Patients and families may each benefit from mutual support.

CONTINUITY OF CARE/DISCHARGE PLANNING
- Institute behavioral and pharmacological treatments. (Depression and substance abuse may become complications; depression responds to tricyclic anti-depressants.)

BIBLIOGRAPHY

American Psychiatric Association (APA). (1994). *Diagnostic and statistical manual of mental disorders.* (4th ed.). Washington, DC: APA.

North American Nursing Diagnosis Association (NANDA). (1992). *Definitions and classification.* St. Louis, MO: NANDA.

Pender, N. J. (1987). *Health promotion in nursing practice* (2nd ed.). Norwalk, CT: Appleton & Lange.

Task Force on *DSM-IV*, American Psychiatric Association (APA). (1991). *DSM-IV options book: Work in progress.* Washington, DC: APA.

Whitley, G. (1991). Ritualistic behavior: Breaking the cycle. *Journal of Psychosocial Nursing, 29*(10), 31–35.

Zinbarg, R., Barlow, D., Brown, T., & Hertz, R. (1992). Cognitive behavioral approaches to the nature and treatment of anxiety disorders. *Annual Review of Psychology, 43,* 235–267.

$\mathscr{P}$OSTTRAUMATIC STRESS DISORDER

Joan Norris, PhD, RN

Posttraumatic Stress Disorder (PTSD) occurs in response to a highly distressing event that is beyond the customary range of most human experiences and evokes feelings of terror and helplessness. Events might include seeing another person killed or tortured, destruction of one's home by natural disaster, rape, and war. The event may be relived in dreams or flashbacks; the person may experience avoidance, amnesia or emotional numbing, and anxiety-related symptoms such as insomnia, wariness, and irritability. Future definitions of this disorder may be more specific in identifying the nature of stressors and the duration (currently 1 month) of time between the trauma and a diagnosis of PTSD if the symptoms continue.

ETIOLOGIES
- Exposure to an exceptionally stressful experience that threatened the life or physical integrity of self or others
- Possible interaction of individual vulnerability, intensity of the trauma, and the support milieu

CLINICAL MANIFESTATIONS
- The extraordinary event is
  - repeatedly reexperienced in nightmares or flashbacks; a sense of reliving the event can include illusions or hallucinations; there may be emotional distress.
  - associated with stimuli that resemble elements of the event or occur on anniversary dates.
- Avoidance behaviors include any of the following:
  - efforts to forget related thoughts and feelings associated with the event
  - amnesia about aspects of the event
  - psychic numbing

–detachment and restricted feelings toward others
- Patient may also experience
  –ongoing sleep disturbances.
  –irritability or impulsiveness.
  –excessive wariness.
  –difficulties in concentration.
  –physical responses of anxiety in situations related to the trauma. (These symptoms were not present prior to the event.)
- There may be associated anxiety, depression, and/or substance abuse.

CLINICAL/DIAGNOSTIC FINDINGS
(None)

▶ NURSING DIAGNOSIS: *Posttrauma Response*

Related To
- Disaster
- War
- Epidemic
- Rape
- Assault
- Torture
- Catastrophic accident

Defining Characteristics
- Reexperience of the trauma in flashbacks, intrusive thoughts, nightmares
- Verbalization about survivor guilt or behavior required for survival
- Emotional numbness, vague recall, constricted affect
- Altered life-style (self-destructiveness, substance abuse)
- Poor impulse control, explosiveness
- Difficulty with interpersonal relationships

Patient Outcomes
Patient will increasingly
- understand the nature and treatment of PTSD.
- recall memories of the traumatic event with reduced anxiety.
- experience feelings and positive relationships with significant others.

Nursing Interventions	Rationales
Assess the nature and extent of posttrauma symptoms and assess for coexisting substance abuse and/or depression.	Patient is helped in identifying and naming the problems and exploring situations that evoke distress through the assessment.
Educate patient about the condition and treatment.	Education provides participation and fosters a sense of control and optimism.

Nursing Interventions	Rationales
Teach anxiety reduction skills such as relaxation training and imagery.	Patient is able to reduce tension when recalling or reexperiencing the traumatic event as well as to reduce general anxiety.
Teach cognitive skills of thought stopping and cognitive restructuring (e.g., valuing the strengths that led to coping and surviving).	Mastering relaxation skills and techniques for interrupting noxious thoughts and replacing them with acceptable ones fosters a sense of control.
Educate and support family.	Promoting understanding of the patient's responses and assisting the family to be supportive strengthens family relationships.
Identify available support groups for patient and family (e.g., Women against Violence, Vietnam Veterans, and others).	Self-help and support groups provide understanding, mutual aid, and problem solving.
Foster communication and exploration of feelings.	A climate of acceptance will encourage the patient to get in touch with and integrate feelings, gaining comfort in expressing them.
Adapt communication to the patient's anxiety level.	Misinterpretation due to severe anxiety is prevented.

▶ **NURSING DIAGNOSIS:** *Rape-Trauma Syndrome (Compound and Silent Reactions)*

Related To disorganization and vulnerability following forced sexual penetration against one's will and consent.

Defining Characteristics

Compound Reaction
- Emotional reactions: fear, humiliation, self-blame, anger
- Physical symptoms: muscle tension, sleep disturbance, gastrointestinal and urinary problems
- Substance abuse as self-medication for distress
- Life-style changes: change of residence, efforts to cope with nightmares and phobic reactions

Silent Reaction
- Abrupt changes in relationships with men
- Increase in nightmares
- Stuttering; blocking of associations
- Physical distress
- Pronounced changes in sexual behavior
- No verbalization that rape occurred
- Sudden onset of phobic symptoms

Patient Outcomes
Patient will increasingly
- experience reduced physical and emotional distress.
- receive and utilize social support.
- regain feelings of mastery and control in life situations.

Nursing Interventions	Rationales
Acute Care	
Perform physical assessment, documentation, and treatment of injuries in a sensitive, accepting, gentle manner.	An understanding atmosphere assures physical status, protects evidence, and maintains attitude of respect and concern for victim.
Assure safety and support for patient during and following (ER) dismissal.	Patients may be incapable of decision making and/or be too frightened to return home or stay alone.
Provide support information and/or assistance from community resources for rape counseling and support.	Encouraging and facilitating mutual aid and assistance promote emotional healing.
Reorganization Phase	
Encourage and accept expression of feelings and thoughts.	It is important to convey acceptance of patient's individualized responses.
Engage in individual or group work to express and resolve feelings and issues.	Mutual support and acceptance permit exploration and working through of responses.
Encourage goal setting and activities to resume a sense of control and self-confidence in life.	Activities should be prioritized and timed to assure success and promote feelings of accomplishment and competence.

CONTINUITY OF CARE/DISCHARGE PLANNING

- Provide for early effective treatment to reduce chronicity and the severity of impairments in relationships and role performance. (Brief hospitalization may be needed to lower risk for depression, suicide, and substance abuse.)
- Encourage outpatient therapy.
- Refer patient and/or family members to support groups.
- Provide symptomatic treatment of severe anxiety and depression (short-term benzodiazepines and tricyclic antidepressants) Propranodol (beta blocker) prn (because of the high risk for substance abuse associated with benzodiazepines).

BIBLIOGRAPHY

American Psychiatric Association (APA). (1994). *Diagnostic and statistical manual of mental disorders* (4th ed.). Washington, DC: APA.

Coughlan, K., & Parkin, C (1987). Women partners of Vietnam vets. *Journal of Psychosocial Nursing, 25*(10), 25–27.

Mejo, S. (1987). Post-traumatic stress disorder: An overview of three etiological variables and psychopharmacologic treatment. *Nurse Practitioner, 15*(8), 41–45.

North American Nursing Diagnosis Association (NANDA). (1992). *Definitions and classification.* St. Louis, MO: NANDA.

Task Force on *DSM-IV,* American Psychiatric Association (APA). (1991). *DSM-IV options book: Work in progress.* Washington, DC: APA.

GENERALIZED ANXIETY DISORDER

Joan Norris, PhD, RN

The characteristic feature of Generalized Anxiety Disorder (GAD) is a long-standing tendency to worry excessively and unrealistically about more than one aspect of life, such as children, finances, and/or role performance. Observable signs and symptoms include motor tension and fatigue; central nervous system hyperactivity including increased vital signs, diaphoresis, and gastrointestinal disturbance; and wariness/hypervigilance with difficulties in concentrating, sleep disturbance, and irritability for 6 months or more. To assist in distinguishing between obsessions and generalized anxiety, the term "unrealistic worries" may be dropped from GAD and "ego dystonic" added to the description of obsessions.

ETIOLOGIES
- May follow a Major Depressive Episode
- Not associated with organic factors such as hyperthyroidism or excess use of caffeine
- Onset most common in young adulthood
- Possibly, slightly more common in women

CLINICAL MANIFESTATIONS
- Unrealistic, excessive worries (6 months or more in duration involving two or more areas of life)
- Motor tension (tremors and/or shakiness, restlessness, muscle tension and soreness, fatigue)
- Central nervous system hyperactivity (dyspnea, tachycardia, diaphoresis, dry mouth, vertigo, gastrointestinal distress, frequent urination, difficulty swallowing)
- Wariness, vigilance (feeling edgy, jumpy, difficulty concentrating, irritability and sleep disturbances)

- Common consequences of GAD include loss of morale and confidence and social anxiety

CLINICAL/DIAGNOSTIC FINDINGS
- None (depression or unrelated panic disorders may be present)

▶ NURSING DIAGNOSIS
(See Anxiety, page 106.)

CONTINUITY OF CARE/DISCHARGE PLANNING
- Engage in outpatient treatment that emphasizes anxiety management (i.e., progressive relaxation and cognitive-behavioral strategies)

BIBLIOGRAPHY
American Psychiatric Association (APA). (1994). *Diagnostic and statistical manual of mental disorders* (4th ed.). Washington, DC: APA.

Butler, G., Fennell, M., Robson, P., & Gelder, M. (1991). Comparison of behavior therapy and cognitive behavior therapy in the treatment of generalized anxiety disorder. *Journal of Consulting and Clinical Psychology, 59*(1), 176–175.

Task Force on *DSM-IV*, American Psychiatric Association (APA). (1991). *DSM-IV options book: Work in progress.* Washington, DC: APA.

Somatoform Disorders

Marga Simon Coler, EdD, RN, CS, CTN, FAAN

Somatoform disorders are characterized by physical symptoms that suggest a medical condition but are not fully explained medically nor by the effects of a substance or by another mental disorder. The symptoms cause social, occupational, or other functional impairments. There is clinical distress. Neither physical nor laboratory findings can be demonstrated. The *Diagnostic and Statistical Manual* (DSM-IV) classifies Somatization Disorder, Undifferentiated Somatoform Disorder, Conversion Disorder, Pain Disorder, Hypochondriasis, Body Dysmorphic Disorder, Pain Disorder, Undifferentiated Somatoform Disorder, and Somatoform Disorder not Otherwise Classified within the major category of Somatoform Disorders. Two of the most commonly encountered, Hypochondriasis and Conversion Disorders, will be developed to illustrate Somatoform Disorders.

The Somatoform Nursing Syndrome is represented by the human response patterns (HRPs) choosing, exchanging, feeling, and perceiving as follows:

HRP	Nursing Diagnosis	Related To
Choosing	Ineffective individual coping	Inability to cope with problems in culturally appropriate manner due to unconscious psychological discomfort
Exchanging	High risk for disuse syndrome	Inability to use affected part due to severe anxiety
Feeling	Pain	Fear of psychological origin
Perceiving	Powerlessness	Inability to consciously relate fear with psychologically caused somatic manifestations

Nursing Interventions	Rationales
Refer for insight-oriented group therapy.	Insight creates an awareness from feedback by group members and therapist, which permits individual to focus on psychogenic origin of pain.
Initiate transactional analysis (TA) therapy.	Transactional analysis teaches strategies of empowerment and creates an awareness of psychodynamic forces which serves to enhance self-control.
Initiate gestalt therapy.	Gestalt therapy provides a safe environment for acting out the displacement toward a goal of experiencing the psychological forces which are the origin of the pain.
Involve in psychodrama.	Psychodrama provides a safe atmosphere for exploring appropriate substitution of symptoms.
Utilize behavior modification.	Behavior modification provides a mechanism for substituting acceptable for unacceptable coping behavior.
Involve in support groups.	Support groups provide support (concern) and feedback from individuals who are experiencing similar problems.

Nursing Interventions	Rationales
Initiate biofeedback.	Biofeedback provides control over obsessive thinking through the conscious selection of body-regulating mechanisms.
Institute psychopharmacological therapy.	There is often underlying anxiety and depression which must be addressed before other interventions can become effective.

$\mathcal{C}$ONVERSION DISORDER

Marga Simon Coler, EdD, RN, CS, CTN, FAAN

$\mathbf{C}$onversion Disorder is a loss or alteration in voluntary motor or sensory functioning that seems to suggest psychological factors. The symptoms are preceded by stressors or conflict. The symptoms are not intentional, nor can they be explained physiologically. The mechanisms that explain what the affected individual derives from this disorder seem to serve as primary and secondary gains. In realizing a primary gain, the individual is able to keep the conflict or need out of awareness; therefore the symptoms have a symbolic effect such as blindness, keeping the individual from acknowledging an especially psychological painful event that he or she witnessed. The mechanism for secondary gain keeps a person from participating in an event or assuming responsibilities that are psychologically feared. This might be exemplified by an unexplainable paralysis before participating in combat. Subtypes are: With Motor Symptoms or Deficit, With Sensory Symptoms or Deficit, With Seizures or Convulsions, With Mixed Presentation.

ETIOLOGIES
- A highly stressful situation
- Knowledge of or exposure to persons with the real (or conversion) impairment

CLINICAL MANIFESTATIONS
- Symptoms affect voluntary motor or sensory activity and mimic a medical condition (most common impairments are manifested by symptoms of blindness, paralysis, paresthesia, seizures, and disturbances in coordination).
- The symptoms are not feigned.
- The symptoms are preceded by conflicts or a period of high stress.
- The impairment cannot be explained by a physical or by laboratory examination.

- The impairment causes social, occupational, physical, and emotional distress.
- The symptoms appear suddenly during a period of stress.
- At times there exists an incongruent lack of concern toward the impairment ("la belle indifference").
- There is no conscious awareness of intentionality of symptom production.
- There is impairment of social and occupational functioning.

CLINICAL/DIAGNOSTIC FINDINGS
- Alteration in physical functioning with no clinical/diagnostic findings

▶ NURSING DIAGNOSIS: *High Risk for Personal Identity Disturbance*

Risk Factors
- Physical signs and symptoms that cannot be validated by physical or laboratory exams
- Uncertainty
- Fear
- Subjective distress
- Self-doubt
- Impairment of social, academic and/or occupational functioning
- Identity confusion
- Depersonalization

Patient Outcomes
Patient will
- experience self-awareness through feelings and perceptions.
- overcome the physical handicap and resume a normal lifestyle.

Nursing Interventions	Rationales
Engage patient in formulating care plan.	Active participation in plan of care will enhance self-esteem.
Engage patient in monitoring progress.	Active participation will help achieve a sense of progress.
Conduct a thorough physical assessment including laboratory examination.	A thorough physical assessment supported by normal laboratory findings will rule out a physiological cause for the disorder, thereby not sanctioning assumption of sick role.
Assist patient in identifying recent stressors through one-on-one psychotherapy.	By identifying recent stressors, the patient may begin to clarify the role of self in relation to that stressor.

Nursing Interventions	Rationales
Teach assertiveness strategies.	A sense of autonomy will be perceived through increasingly assertive behavior. Autonomy enhances self-esteem.
Change from directive to nondirective leadership style with increasingly assertive patient behavior.	As client begins to achieve a sense of self, autonomous acts must be encouraged and strengthened.

▶ NURSING DIAGNOSIS: *Sensory/Perceptual Alterations (Kinesthetic)*

Related To an intense preoccupation that one has a serious disease, intrapsychic conflicts, and psychosocial stressors.

Defining Characteristics
- Inappropriate bodily responses (signs/symptoms)
- Anxiety
- Fear
- Pain
- Misinterpretation of normal bodily functions
- Perceiving in physical instead of emotional terms

Patient Outcomes
Patient will
- decrease somatic complaints.
- demonstrate a recognition of and insight into somatic complaints.
- identify source of anxiety.
- modify coping patterns.

Nursing Interventions	Rationales
Perform comprehensive physical and laboratory examinations.	Normal physical and laboratory findings help rule out physical pathology.
Initiate one-on-one psychotherapy.	A one-on-one relationship enhances trust.
Initiate behavior modification therapy.	Behavior therapy has been reported to be successful in helping to restore sensations and perceptions of stimuli.

▶ NURSING DIAGNOSIS: *Ineffective Individual Coping*

Related To
- Psychological conflicts or needs
- Denial of expression of an unacceptable drive
- Conversion of this drive into a somatic symptom (symbolic expression)
- Unconscious mechanisms of repression and conversion

Defining Characteristics
- Inability to meet role expectations
- Inappropriate use of unconscious defense mechanisms
- Self-destructive behavior
- Occasional inappropriate reaction to conversion
- Alteration in meeting role expectations

Patient Outcomes
Patient will
- resume preincident adaptive coping patterns.
- learn new adaptive coping behaviors to stressor.

Nursing Interventions	Rationales
Provide mechanism for expression of fears and anxieties.	Allowing patient to express the fear and anxieties helps patient to experience feelings and emotions associated with that event toward an end of converting maladaptive coping mechanisms to adaptive ones.
Assist patient in identifying adaptive coping mechanisms to identified stressor.	The identification of adaptive coping mechanisms might bring about changes in coping patterns.
Provide supportive one-to-one psychotherapy.	A trusting relationship will provide support during the reconversion of maladaptive coping to adaptive patterns.

▶ NURSING DIAGNOSIS: *Spiritual Distress*

Related To
- A disruption of an important life principle
- Challenge of value system
- High psychosocial stress situation

Defining Characteristics
- Expressed concern over violation of an important life principle
- Verbalization of conflict
- Alteration in mood
- Lack of concern over conversion symptoms

Patient Outcomes
Patient will
- explain relationship of his or her life to event in culturally adaptive terms.
- redefine life principle to stressful event.
- demonstrate acceptance of his or her role in stressful event.
- reconvert conversion symptoms.

Nursing Interventions	Rationales
Engage in individual psychotherapy: 1. Encourage verbalization of conflict with values. 2. Reinforce reality. 3. Explore alternative options for adapting life principles to reality. 4. Encourage adaptive, independent decision making.	Because of psychogenic origin of disorder, many professionals in psychiatry feel that only psychotherapy would be expected to provide lasting benefits. 1. Verbalization gives therapist insight that may be reflected to patient's value system. 2. Reality therapy is aimed at changing maladaptive psychosocial perceptions. 3. Alternative options may help patient give up need for primary and/or secondary gain in order to modify maladaptive value system. 4. Decisions relating to values must be made by the affected individual to help alleviate spiritual distress.
Engage patient in support group related to the psychosocial stressor.	Supportive group therapy may help modify a rigid value system when patient can relate to similar spiritual struggles in others.
Initiate consultation with clergy prn.	Spiritual distress is often tied to religious mores which might be modified through enlightenment by talking with a specialist in the patient's religion.

CONTINUITY OF CARE/DISCHARGE PLANNING
- Utilize crisis intervention strategies as necessary.
- Provide for pharmacological intervention prn.
- Refer to long-term supportive individual or group psychotherapy.

BIBLIOGRAPHY
American Psychiatric Association (APA). (1994). *Diagnostic and statistical manual of mental disorders* (4th ed.). Washington, DC: APA.

Burgess, A. (1990). *Psychiatric nursing in the hospital and the community.* Norwalk, CT: Appleton & Lange.

Goldman, H. (1988). *General psychiatry.* Norwalk, CT: Appleton & Lange.

Koneazny, K. (1992). Coping, impaired, individual. In K. Gettrust & P. Brabec (Eds.), *Nursing diagnosis in clinical practice.* Albany, NY: Delmar.

MacFarland, G., & McFarlane, E. (1989). *Nursing diagnosis and intervention.* St. Louis, MO: Mosby.

Simsandl, G., & VandeVusse, L. (1992). Sensory perception, altered. In K. Gettrust & P. Brabec (Eds.), *Nursing diagnosis in clinical practice.* Albany, NY: Delmar.

Task Force on *DSM-IV*, American Psychiatric Association (APA). (1993). *DSM-IV draft criteria.* Washington, DC: APA.

Task Force on *DSM-IV*, American Psychiatric Association (APA). (1991). *DSM-IV options book: Work in progress.* Washington, DC: APA.

Valentin, C. (1992). Personal identity disturbance. In K. Gettrust & P. Brabec (Eds.), *Nursing diagnosis in clinical practice.* Albany, NY: Delmar.

VandeVusse, L., & Simsandl, G. (1992). Sensory perception, altered. In K. Gettrust & P. Brabec (Eds.), *Nursing diagnosis in clinical practice.* Albany, NY: Delmar.

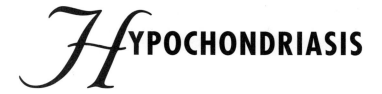

HYPOCHONDRIASIS

Marga Simon Coler, EdD, RN, CS, CTN, FAAN

Hypochondriasis, a persistent preoccupation of at least 6 months with fears of having a serious disease, stems from a misinterpretation of bodily symptoms. This occurs despite reassurance to the contrary, based on thorough medical evaluation. The preoccupation causes impairment in all areas of functioning (occupational, social, etc.). There is marked psychological distress (APA, 1994).

ETIOLOGIES
- Past experience with true organic disease in oneself or a family member
- Psychosocial stressors
- Anxiety, depression, and Obsessive-Compulsive Personality Disorders
- Average age of onset, 20–30 years

CLINICAL MANIFESTATIONS
- Preoccupation with fear or idea that one has a serious disease
- Persistent preoccupation despite appropriate reassurance
- Lack of findings on physical examination or laboratory tests
- Failure to develop the feared disease
- Duration for at least 6 months
- A transcultural malady

Clinical Clip

It is a well-known fact that Eastern and Latin cultures tend to develop somatic symptoms to stress-related situations. This is different from hypochondriasis.

CLINICAL/DIAGNOSTIC FINDINGS
• Hypochondriasis is characterized by an absence of clinical/diagnostic findings

▶ NURSING DIAGNOSIS: *Anxiety*

Related To a fear or idea that one has a serious disease despite contrary laboratory and medical evidence.

Defining Characteristics
• Tension
• Apprehension
• Helplessness (increased, painful, persistent)
• Uncertainty
• Fright
• Distress
• Confusion
• Inadequacy
• Change in sleeping habits
• Change in eating habits
• Change in elimination habits
• Distractibility
• Difficulty expressing self verbally
• Irritability
• Nausea/vomiting
• Indecisiveness
• Tachycardia
• Hyperventilation

Patient Outcomes
Patient will
• verbally and behaviorally demonstrate a decrease in anxiety.
• assume control over signs and symptoms.
• utilize adaptive coping strategies (relaxation, biofeedback, reality testing, problem solving, leisure activities).

Nursing Interventions	Rationales
Conduct a thorough physical and laboratory examination.	A thorough assessment rules out physiological causes of symptoms.
Conduct a thorough nursing history.	A thorough assessment provides data for interventions.
Review and discuss diagnosis with patient.	Insight is essential for effective treatment.
Plan treatment with patient.	Successful intervention is dependent on patient input.
Rule out major depression and anxiety.	Somatic complaints are prevalent in depression and anxiety, but require other interventions.

Nursing Interventions	Rationales
Consider chemical intervention for underlying symptomatology of depression and anxiety.	Medication may be indicated and should be prescribed if helpful in controlling symptoms toward an end of gaining insight into hypochondriasis.
Plan psychotherapeutic intervention.	Psychotherapy will help to identify sources of underlying depression and anxiety.
Teach self-control strategies.	Self-control can decrease anxiety.
Teach problem-solving strategies.	Problem-solving strategies provide adaptive ways of resolving conflicts, which will, in turn, decrease anxiety.
Teach strategies for developing an unencumbering, daily routine to avoid confusion.	Thinking in a state of anxiety is diffuse and requires a routine to avoid confusion.

Clinical Clip

Thinking and concentration are difficult for those who are experiencing anxiety. A highly structured routine helps to direct thought and actions.

▶ NURSING DIAGNOSIS: *Fear*

Related To a feeling that one has a serious disease.

Defining Characteristics
- Identification of object of fear
- Apprehension
- Avoidance behavior
- Guilt, shame
- Heightened imagination
- Intelligent, intentional action toward object of fear
- Psychophysiological changes
- Self- and other-directed aggression
- Hypervigilance

Patient Outcomes
Patient will
- identify object of fear.
- assume control over the object of fear.
- put fear into a proper perspective.
- identify significance of object of fear relative to life's goal.

- utilize culturally appropriate coping skills.
- identify and utilize appropriate past coping mechanisms in dealing with the object of fear.
- master and utilize new coping mechanisms in dealing with the object of fear.
- identify and link with past and present support systems for dealing with the object of fear.

Nursing Interventions	Rationales
Assess background of sense of fear.	Assessment helps determine if the emotion of fear is based on reality, misinformation, or classical conditioning.
Assess the intensity of fear relative to age, sex, socioeconomic class, and ethnicity.	Responses to an object of fear may be determined by these factors.
Determine extent of victimization by fear production techniques by external sources.	Fear-inducing techniques are frequently employed as part of conscious attempts to muster commitment to groups or causes or to create divisiveness among populations.
Initiate short-term psychotherapy.	Psychotherapy helps client identify object of the fear.
Examine the significance of the object of fear.	Such insight helps to understand the sensed reality. Frequently, the greater the significance, the greater the distortion.
Identify the fear-expressing mechanisms.	The emotional response to fear mechanisms may be rational or irrational. It is important to identify both responses to mobilize appropriate coping mechanisms.
Factor out components of the feared object.	Factoring out helps minimize the whole, thereby permitting the prioritization of significant parts.
Enhance psychic repetition of feared event.	Psychic repetition achieves belated mastery of emotions related to the event.
Initiate assertiveness training.	Assertiveness helps client confront the object of fear which may have

Nursing Interventions	Rationales
	supressed the feelings which produce normal assertiveness.
Aid in separating beliefs about the object of fear.	Undesirable emotional consequences from the actual object of fear can often be traced to irrational beliefs.
Aid in the separation of emotional, cognitive, perceptual, and behavioral responses to fear.	The separation of response components aids in coping with the object of fear in a rational manner.
Assist in channeling fear-producing energy into creative fear-resolving strategies.	Maladaptive emotions can be channeled into creativity through the use of insight and education.
Educate toward goal of gaining unbiased knowledge about object of fear.	Knowledge corrects misconceptions.
Teach the physiological response reactions to fear.	Knowledge about the mechanisms of physiological responses helps to maintain control over them.
Teach how fear is expressed and communicated through symbols and the public media within a culture.	Knowledge about the strategies of fear production and their effect on the human organism will provide insight into irrational emotions, feelings, and behaviors toward the object of fear.
Consider systematic desensitization.	Systematic desensitization is easy to comprehend, mandates client participation, and has proven to be effective.
Relate cultural concepts to conditions under which fear arises.	The origin of fear may be different from one culture to another. In order to respond to the object of fear appropriately, the feelings and insights must be culturally appropriate.

▶ NURSING DIAGNOSIS: *High Risk for Personal Identity Disturbance*

Risk Factors
- Erroneous beliefs about self
- Physical signs and symptoms that cannot be validated by physical or laboratory exams

- Uncertainty
- Frustration
- Fear
- Anxiety

- Subjective distress
- Self-doubt
- Impulsivity
- Oppositional thinking (to community, family, etc.)
- Impairment of social, academic and/or occupational functioning
- Helplessness
- Identity confusion

- Identity diffusion
- Narcissism
- Loss of sense of time
- Depersonalization
- Lack of empathy
- Lack of intimacy
- Low self-esteem
- Low self-concept
- Sense of alienation

Patient Outcomes
Patient will
- attain self-realization.
- experience self-awareness through feelings and perceptions.
- make choices based on expressed values.
- maintain relationships with significant others, peers, superordinates, and subordinates for 6 months.

Nursing Interventions	Rationales
Engage patient in formulating care plan.	Active participation in plan of care will enhance self-esteem.
Engage patient in monitoring progress.	Active participation will help achieve a sense of progress.
Assist patient in identifying roles.	Role clarification helps patient attain a sense of authenticity.
Teach assertiveness.	A sense of autonomy will be perceived through increasingly assertive behavior. Autonomy enhances self-esteem.
Change from directive to nondirective leadership style with increasingly assertive patient behavior.	As client begins to achieve a sense of self, autonomous acts must be encouraged and strengthened.

▶ NURSING DIAGNOSIS: *Sensory/Perceptual Alterations (Kinesthetic)*

Related To an intense preoccupation that one has a serious disease.

Defining Characteristics
- Inappropriate bodily responses (signs/symptoms)
- Anxiety
- Fear

- Pain
- Excessive "shopping" for health care provider
- Augmentation and amplification of normal bodily sensations
- Misinterpretation of normal bodily functions
- Perceiving in physical instead of emotional terms

Patient Outcomes

Patient will
- decrease somatic complaints.
- demonstrate a recognition of and insight into somatic complaints.
- identify source of anxiety.
- modify coping patterns.

Nursing Interventions	Rationales
Establish a one-to-one contract.	A one-to-one relationship enhances trust.
Perform comprehensive physical and laboratory examinations.	Normal physical and laboratory findings help rule out physical pathology.
Initiate insight-oriented therapy.	Insight assists patient to recognize and deal with the etiology of alterations in sensororium and perceptions, which will in turn help to alter the behavior.
Initiate behavior modification therapy.	Insight alone generally does not help to alleviate symptoms.

CONTINUITY OF CARE/DISCHARGE PLANNING
- Evaluate periodically for depression which may cloak anxiety.
- Provide for pharmacological intervention as needed.
- Refer to long-term psychotherapy (weekly to bi-weekly to monthly).

BIBLIOGRAPHY

American Psychiatric Association (APA). (1994). *Diagnostic and statistical manual of mental disorders* (4th ed.). Washington, DC: APA.

Burgess, A. (1990). *Psychiatric nursing in the hospital and the community.* Norwalk, CT: Appleton & Lange.

Coler, M. (1992). Fear. In K. Gettrust & P. Brabec (Eds.), *Nursing diagnosis in clinical practice: Guides for care planning.* Albany, NY: Delmar.

Greenson, R. (1986). *The technique and practice of psychotherapy.* New York: International Universities Press.

Haber, J., Mc Mahon, A., Price-Hoskins, A., & Sideleau, B. (1992). *Psychiatric nursing.* St. Louis, MO: Mosby-Year Book.

MacFarland, G., & McFarlane, E. (1989). *Nursing diagnosis and intervention.* St. Louis, MO: Mosby.

Patterson, C. (1986). *Theories of counseling and psychotherapy.* New York: Harper & Row.

Stuart, G., & Sundeen, S. (1991). *Principles and practice of psychiatric nursing.* St. Louis, MO: Mosby Year-Book.

Task Force on *DSM-IV*, American Psychiatric Association (APA). (1991). *DSM-IV options book: Work in progress.* Washington, DC: APA.

Task Force on *DSM-IV*, American Psychiatric Association (APA). (1993). *DSM-IV draft criteria.* Washington, DC: APA.

Vincent, K. (1992). Anxiety. In K. Gettrust & P. Brabec (Eds.), *Nursing diagnosis in clinical practice: Guides for care planning.* Albany, NY: Delmar.

Walker, J. (1985). *Essentials of clinical psychiatry.* Philadelphia, PA: Lippincott.

Dissociative Disorders

Regina Sebree, MS, RN, ARNP

Dissociation is a psychophysiological process in which there is a separation of emotions, thoughts, and/or behaviors from the patient's current stream of consciousness. The functions of personal identity, memory, and consciousness, which usually act in unison to define the "self" for a person, are altered to protect the ego from overwhelming material. Persons cannot take flight or fight to cope with overwhelming trauma, so they disengage their feelings into a separate consciousness. Dissociation is a survival coping mechanism and occurs on a continuum. At one end are common episodes of dissociation, such as daydreaming, "tuning out" conversation, or highway hypnosis. At the other end of the continuum are major Dissociative Disorders such as Dissociative Fugue and Dissociative Identity Disorders. Although the cause of the diseases is unknown, suggested etiologies include innate capacity to dissociate, severe chronic, unpredictable sexual/or physical abuse, and defense against conflicted affects. These diseases are not due to substance abuse or a co-occurring medical condition. Patients may present with an inability to recall events and two or more distinct personalities which control behavior, including individual ways of perceiving, relating, and acting within the environment. Three instruments are used to measure dissociative experiences: Dissociative Experience Scale (DES), Dissociative Disorders Interview Scale (DDIS), and the Structured Clinical Interview for

DSM-IV Dissociative Disorders. The human response patterns (HRPs) which identify the syndrome are perceiving and relating.

HRP	Nursing Diagnosis	Related To
Perceivng	Sensory/perceptual alterations	Attempt by the internal psyche to cope with extreme forms of abuse
Relating	Impaired social interaction	Past history of abusive relationships and altered states of consciousness

Nursing Interventions	Rationales
Initiate individual psychotherapy.	One-to-one psychotherapy assists in reality testing, working through past traumatic experiences (identifying the perpertrators and helping to heal the self-esteem); provides a consistent, available, and therapeutic relationship as a model for redoing traumas with others in the past; and helps in identifying the different "alters" within the psyche and begins to communicate with each.
Initiate milieu therapy.	Milieu therapy is provided when there is a danger for harm to self or others; it enables learning of social skills in a protected and therapeutic environment.

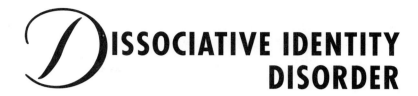

ISSOCIATIVE IDENTITY DISORDER

Regina Sebree, MS, RN, ARNP

The *Diagnostic and Statistical Manual* (DSM-IV) changes *Multiple Personality Disorder* (MPD) to *Dissociative Identity Disorder,* which deemphasizes the movie portrayal of the disorder and more accurately names it. This disorder, once thought to be rare, is now believed to affect 10% of the general population. Approximately 200 cases were reported in the literature before 1980. By 1986 an estimated 6,000 cases had been diagnosed in North America alone.

ETIOLOGIES
- Abuse or severe childhood trauma seem to be precursors.

CLINICAL MANIFESTATIONS
- Presence of two or more distinct personality states that take control of the person's behavior
- Inability to recall important personal information not due to substance abuse or a medical condition

CLINICAL/DIAGNOSTIC FINDINGS
- Prior treatment failure
- Multiple psychiatric diagnoses

▶ NURSING DIAGNOSIS: *Personal Identity Disturbance*
Related To
- Use of dissociation to cope with overwhelming trauma
- Severe chronic childhood sexual and/or physical abuse

Defining Characteristics
- Loss of time or inability to account for time
- Feelings of unreality
- Finding oneself in an unfamiliar place
- Flashbacks
- Nightmares
- Marked changes in style of dress, grooming, and mannerisms
- Change in speech: rate, pitch, accent, and loudness
- Rapid blinking, tics, and twitches
- Changes in personal habits and preferences, i.e., smoking and taste in music
- Making self-references in the plural or third person

Patient Outcomes
Patient will
- gain control over feelings and behaviors that prompted admission.
- begin to join with disruptive alters in the therapy process.
- have learned to coexist with alters for the good of the whole.

Nursing Interventions	Rationales
Assess and explore expectations of hospitalization.	The hospital is sometimes seen as a place to "rest" or "to forget" or patients may experience the hospital as a place of retraumatization.
Assess knowledge of the diagnosis.	Nursing interventions depend on the patients' knowledge of the diagnosis and what phase of treatment they are in. They may not know any of their alters or they may know all of them.
Assess the alters: names, ages, and characteristics.	Knowing the alters assists the nurse in understanding the psychological needs of the patient by knowing the function the alter has with the person.
Assess who are the helpful alters in a crisis.	Internal self-helpers (ISHs) are knowledgeable about the individual in an objective manner and function in the system primarily as helpers.
Use caution in making any physical contact.	Physical contact has been experienced as abusive, not comforting or nurturing.

Nursing Interventions	Rationales
Maintain clear boundaries.	Personal boundaries have been invaded most of their lives, and patients therefore do not always understand helpful boundaries. They may attempt to intrude into the nurse's personal life. Boundaries help to maintain safety in the relationship.
Assign to a private room if possible.	A private room provides a safe place to retreat if patient feels overwhelmed.
Be aware of transference and countertransference issues.	The nurse usually experiences excitement and is overinvested in the beginning of the relationship, which as time passes, changes to a sense of being drained.
Set the expectation to attend all milieu meetings. Allow them to choose their level of participation.	Some do not tolerate milieu meetings and groups well but need to attend as much as possible to avoid the risk of isolation from the community.
Encourage to acknowledge what they do and do not remember.	Gaps in memory have been covered as a way of coping with his or her dissociative identity.
Allow to sleep with back to a wall if patient feels safer. Leave a night light on.	Patients feel safer with their backs to the wall or a light on, probably related to the abuse.
Discuss their responsibility for the behaviors of the total person.	Continually encourage wholeness in the person.
Empathize with the frustration of taking responsibility for all behaviors and encourage to pursue knowing the alters.	The alters are fragments of the person.
Ask to look inside and check it out with the other parts of the self if patient denies a behavior others observed. Believe the alter that is present and denying the behavior.	The personality state denying the behavior was not in control at the time.
Tolerate the need for repetition of instructions regarding unit rules,	The personality state present may not be the personality state the

Nursing Interventions	Rationales
schedules, etc. Ask all alters to listen to instructions or information.	instructions were given to originally.
Call the alters by name if they ask you to do so, but always acknowledge them as part of a whole.	References to the alters as parts of the person encourage integration and discourages further fragmentation.
Accept the patient's reality regardless of the credibility of their memories.	The age at which the dissociation began (as a coping mechanism) usually includes childhood fantasies which may become a part of their memory.
Call out the most helpful personality state in a crisis. Ask: "Who can come and help you now?" "Who can be in control?" "May I speak to that person?" "You need to let _____ come out." "Let us try to help you; have _____ come out." Help patient to relax as the nurse counts from 10 to 1. _____ will come out as you reach 1.	Internal self-helpers function in the personality as helpers. The most helpful person may change as progress is made in therapy.
Develop written contracts and ask all alters for input and to sign. Give the patients a copy of the contract.	Written contracts are useful and tend to be complied with when they are written positively, acknowledging the patient's achievements. Rewards and consequences need to be included.
Limit child alters to their rooms to engage with staff in what to them is age-appropriate behavior.	Child activities done in public may be disruptive to present and future adult relationships with peers.
Be aware that it is difficult to remain in empathic touch across sudden personality changes.	The nurse may be talking to a sad 5-year-old that switches to an angry 12-year-old.
Be aware that personalities often switch when difficult material is anticipated or under discussion.	The alters are a defense.
Identify misperceptions and address matter-of-factly the patients'	Being kept within a hospital unit may be perceived as punishment

Nursing Interventions	Rationales
tendency to distort reality as they perceive staff members as persecutors and themselves as victims.	and the limit setter as an abuser. The holding environment needs to be "good enough," not perfect.
Provide art therapy.	Patients are generally responsive to art therapy as a nonverbal expression.
Initiate movement therapy.	Movement therapy helps to regain a sense of wholeness by experiencing the body and mind in unity.
Engage in cognitive therapy.	Examples of assumptions: Cognitive therapy confronts false assumptions of patient, such as: (a) *Different parts of the self are separate selves;* i.e., I could burn, cut her, and be unaffected myself. I was not abused. (b) *The person is responsible for the abuse.* If I'd been a better child, it wouldn't have happened. I must be bad.
Initiate biofeedback therapy.	Biofeedback therapy helps to regain a sense of wholeness by experiencing the body and mind in unity.
Encourage family therapy.	Family therapy helps to focus on effects on family and the need to establish age-appropriate boundaries between the parents and the children.
Teach the patient to keep a daily journal.	Various alters may write in the journal, depending on who is in control at the time. The journal may be a safer place to communicate with the nurse. It may discourage acting out and be a tool for continuity of experience.
Teach the patient the victim-abuser-rescuer triangle.	When patients understand the triangle, they may be able to look at their behavior more objectively and identify which role they are in.

▶ NURSING DIAGNOSIS: *Posttrauma Response—Spontaneous Abreactions*

Related To severe childhood abuse.

Defining Characteristics
- Flashbacks
- Free-floating anxiety and dread
- Past experienced as present reality
- May verbally cry out

Patient Outcomes
Patient will
- be reanchored in reality so as not to be retraumatized.
- recognize signs of impending abreactions and learn how to contain them until therapy sessions.

Nursing Interventions	Rationales
Remain with the patient.	Posttrauma response is a very confusing and frightening experience. The nurse's presence assists in grounding in reality.
Clarify who the nurse is and where the nurse and patient are [reality orientation].	Reality orientation counteracts the experience of the past as present and helps to ground the patient.
Avoid touching the patient.	Physical contact has been experienced as abusive, not comforting or nurturing.
Assist in learning signals that there is an impending abreaction about to occur. Use journaling flow sheets and feedback from others.	This gives a sense of control and mastery.
Reframe the signals as important messages that patients are giving to themselves and a sign of progress in therapy.	This gives a sense of control that the flashback may be useful in therapy and not just meaningless pain.
Call out an internal helper to contain the memory until a therapy session.	Flashbacks can be experienced as retraumatizing. The ISHs function in the personality system as objective helpers.

Nursing Interventions	Rationales
Provide support when experiencing auditory hallucinations and help focus on reality.	Patients may hear screaming, voices berating, usually the host personality, or commands to be self-destructive. Usually patients describe the voices as going on in their head, which distinguishes them from schizophrenic auditory hallucinations which are generally experienced as coming from outside the person.

▶ **NURSING DIAGNOSIS:** *High Risk for Violence—Directed at Others*

Risk Factors
- An impending or present traumatic, stressful situation
- Specific environmental cues
- Alter identification with the agressor

Nursing Interventions	Rationales
Call out the most helpful personality state when the angry alter is in control to assist in the crisis on the unit.	Internal self-helpers are knowledgeable about the person in an objective manner and function in the system primarily as helpers.
Provide structured and planned use of restraints during psychotherapy sessions: 1. Have patient sign voluntary informed consent to be placed in restraints. 2. Have adequate staff available as patient is being put into restraints as the violent alter may come out. 3. Have nursing staff present during the session to check patient's circulation, etc. 4. Nursing staff need to know what went on during the session to be alert for crises in the coming	Restraints may be needed to allow a violent alter to come out and to protect the patient and staff during the psychotherapy.

Nursing Interventions	Rationales
hours, i.e., an alter threatening to kill another alter.	
Allow the patient a "safe place," if possible, i.e., sitting in a corner or sitting under a desk.	Providing a safe environment gives patient a feeling of being in control of the situation during a flashback experience.

CONTINUITY OF CARE/DISCHARGE PLANNING
- Formulate a contract with patient ensuring own safety.
- Assure continued psychotherapy.
- Establish monitoring mechanism to assure that patient has control over behaviors that precipitated admission.
- Provide linkage with external support system.
- Ascertain that patient continues in outpatient therapy.
- Refer to eating disorder groups or sexual abuse groups as needed.

BIBLIOGRAPHY

Adams, A. (1989). Internal self helpers of persons with multiple personality. *Dissociations, 23,* 138–143.

American Psychiatric Association (APA). (1994). *Diagnostic and statistical manual of mental disorders* (4th ed.). Washington, DC: APA.

Kluft, R. P. (1991). Hospital treatment of multiple personality disorder. *Psychiatric Clinics of North America, 14*(3), 695–719.

North American Nursing Diagnosis Association (NANDA). (1992). *NANDA nursing diagnosis: Definitions and classifications 1992,* St. Louis, MO: NANDA.

Putman, F. W. (1989). *Diagnosis and treatment of multiple personality disorder.* New York: Guilford.

Ross, C. A. (1991). Epidemiology of multiple personality disorder and dissociation. *Psychiatric Clinics of North America, 14*(3), 503–517.

Steele, K., & Colrain, J. (1990). Abreactive work with sexual abuse survivors: Concepts and techniques. In M. Hunger (Ed.), *The sexually abused male* (Vol. 2). Lexington, MA: Lexington Books.

Turkus, J. A. (1991). Psychotherapy and case management for multiple personality disorder. *Psychiatric Clinics of North America, 14*(3), 649–660.

Young, W. C. (1986). Restraints in the treatment of a patient with multiple personality. *American Journal of Psychotherapy, 11*(4), 601–666.

DEPERSONALIZATION DISORDER

Regina Sebree, MS, RN, ARNP

Depersonalization Disorder also involves a disturbance of *identity*. Depersonalization is a phenomenon that involves feelings of being unreal, of watching a movie of oneself, and of numbness in which there is a lack of feelings and yet reality testing is intact. Depersonalization is a *symptom* and a *disorder*. It occurs on a continuum of normal to pathological.

ETIOLOGIES
(Unknown)

CLINICAL MANIFESTATIONS
- Recurring experiences of feelings of unrealness and numbness of feelings.
- Reality testing that remains intact
- Impairment of social and occupational functioning due to dissociative experience and not due to substance abuse or a medical condition is better accounted for by another psychiatric disorder

CLINICAL/DIAGNOSTIC FINDINGS
- Feelings of depersonalization that occur in normal adults during life-threatening trauma, i.e., accidents or extreme stress
- Depersonalization that may occur with a variety of psychiatric disorders such as Posttraumatic Stress Disorder
- Dissociative Identity Disorder or as a separate disorder

▶ NURSING DIAGNOSIS: *Personal Identity Disturbance— Depersonalization*

Related To
- Response to life-threatening dangers, i.e., accidents and serious illnesses
- Response to sexual, physical, and/or cult abuse
- A traumatic memory
- Extreme fatigue
- Sensory deprivation
- Sleep deprivation

Defining Characteristics
- Feelings of strangeness or unreality
- Retention of reality testing
- Numbness, loss of affective response
- Feelings of being disconnected, unreal
- Experience of being outside one's body watching one's self from a distance

Patient Outcomes
Patient will
- verbalize coping strategies to manage stress.
- report a decrease in depersonalization symptoms.
- return to normal social and occupational functioning.

Nursing Interventions	Rationales
Remain with the patient.	Depersonalization is a frightening experience.
Assist to verbalize the experience.	Putting the experience in words assists in gaining mastery and communicating with others.
Explore stressors that precipitated depersonalization and assist in developing other coping strategies.	Identification of concrete stressors helps to gain control.
Teach about depersonalization.	Most patients are fearful of going crazy and need to understand the experience.

CONTINUITY OF CARE/DISCHARGE PLANNING
- Assure a support system outside the hospital.
- Arrange for one-to-one therapy to reinforce positive coping strategies to manage stress.

- Provide supportive therapy on an outpatient basis to assist the patient through other episodes of depersonalization.

BIBLIOGRAPHY

North American Nursing Diagnosis Association (NANDA). (1992). *NANDA nursing diagnosis: Definitions and classifications 1992,* St. Louis, MO: NANDA.

Steinberg, M. (1991). The spectrum of depersonalization: Assessment and treatment. In A. Tasman, & S. M. Goldfinger, (Eds.), *Review of psychiatry #10,* (pp. 223–248). Washington, DC: American Psychiatric Press.

Task Force on *DSM-IV,* American Psychiatric Association (APA). (1993). *DSM-IV draft criteria.* Washington, DC: APA.

Sexual and Gender Identity Disorders

Marga Simon Coler, EdD, RN, CS, CTN, FAAN

In the *Diagnostic and Statistical Manual* (DSM-IV) the Sexual and Gender Identity Disorders are treated as one section. These have been subclassified as Sexual Dysfunctions, Paraphilias, and Gender Identity Disorders and Sexual Disorder not identified elsewhere. All are characterized by considerable distress and interpersonal difficulty between perpetrator, recipient, and cultural norms. Some of the more common ones are discussed. The nursing syndrome is derived from the North American Nursing Diagnosis Association (NANDA) human response patterns (HRPs) valuing, perceiving, relating, and feeling. The syndrome may be defined as a perception of gender identity or sexual function that is not acceptable within the social norms of one's culture. This results in conflicting values regarding sexual relationships, producing feelings of fear and anxiety.

HRP	Nursing Diagnosis	Related To
Valuing	Spiritual distress	Individual values in conflict with culture

HRP	Nursing Diagnosis	Related To
Perceiving	Powerlessness	An uncontrollable urge to engage in maladaptive sexual behavior
	Hopelessness	A subjective state in which there seems no alternative to combating the obsessive sexual feelings
	Chronic low self-esteem	A subjective state in which there exists a subconscious negative self-evaluation about the maladaptive sexual urges
	Personal identity disturbance	An inability to distinguish between the maladaptive and the culturally acceptable self
Relating	Sexual dysfunction	Culturally conflicting value system
	Altered sexuality patterns	Physiological/emotional alterations in body function or structure
	Altered role performance	Disruption in the way one perceives one's sexual role in one's culture
	Impaired social interaction	Cultural/sexual dissonance
Feeling	Fear	Persistent feeling of dread of being hurt, discovered, and/or punished
	Anxiety	An emotional, libidinal, often subconscious tension; sexual distress

Nursing Interventions

Initiate supportive individual psychotherapy.

Rationales

Individual psychotherapy provides insight into the causal relationship between attitudes and behavior, thereby enhancing change from maladaptive to adaptive sexual behavior.

Nursing Interventions	Rationales
Initiate supportive group psychotherapy.	Supportive group therapy provides support from others suffering the same spiritual distress.

SEXUAL DYSFUNCTIONS

Marga Simon Coler, EdD, RN, CS, CTN, FAAN

The sexual dysfunctions are characterized by a disturbance in the processes that characterize the sexual response cycle, or by pain associated with sexual intercourse (APA, 1994). Sexual dysfunctions are lifelong or acquired and generalized or situational. They are subclassified as: Sexual Desire Disorders, Sexual Arousal Disorders, Sexual Aversion Disorders, Orgasmic Disorders, and Sexual Pain Disorders. Each of these are further subclassified in the *Diagnostic and Statistical Manual* (DSM-IV). Sexual dysfunctions are distinguished by four phases: (1) desire (fantasies about and desire to have sexual activity); (2) excitement (a subjective sense of sexual pleasure accompanied by sexual excitement); (3) orgasm (a peaking of sexual pleasure with a subsequent release of sexual tension); and (4) resolution (a sense of well-being accompanied by generalized relaxation). Sexual dysfunctions may occur with a partner or with autostimulation.

ETIOLOGIES
- Emotional tone of a relationship
- Sexual dissatisfaction and/or poor sexual communication
- Anxiety
- Excessively high performance standards
- Real or imagined rejection by partner
- Negative attitude toward sexuality
- Psychopathology

CLINICAL MANIFESTATIONS
- Deficient or absent desires for sexual activities
- Deficient or absent sexual fantasies
- Persistent aversion to genital sexual contact
- Recurrent or persistent failure to attain physiological response of sexual excitement
- Recurrent or persistent absence of, or delay in, achieving an orgasm

- Recurrent or persistent genital pain
- Premature ejaculation in males
- Involuntary, interfering vaginal spasms in female

CLINICAL/DIAGNOSTIC FINDINGS
- A history of sexual abuse or conflict as a child
- Chromosomal abnormality
- Abnormal hormonal level

▶ NURSING DIAGNOSIS: *Sexual Dysfunction*

Related To biopsychosocial factors.

Defining Characteristics
- Actual or perceived sexual limitations
- Persistent psychological or biophysical pain
- Performance anxiety
- Absence of sexual satisfaction
- Intense preoccupation with other life activities

Patient Outcomes
Patient will be able to attain sexual pleasure with partner or upon autostimulation.

Nursing Interventions	Rationales
Assess the existing, intact sexual responses.	The existing responses indicate at what level to begin therapeutic intervention.
Assess for organic, psychological, or social etiological factors.	The type and extent of the etiology will serve as an indicator of what is physically feasible to attain.
Assess relationship between etiological factor(s) and sexual dysfunction.	The relationship between etiology and dysfunction will determine the focus of the psychotherapy.
Assess for attitude of patient and significant other (where indicated) regarding the sexual dysfunction.	The attitude of both parties is instrumental in determining if and what type of psychotherapy is indicated.
Assess for cultural and religious attitudes toward sexual function.	Culture and religious beliefs have a profound influence on sexual behavior and must be considered in the therapeutic plan.

Nursing Interventions	Rationales
Provide anticipatory guidance if the dysfunction is physiologically related.	Knowledge of the repercussion of the effect of physiological changes will aid patient in planning an acceptable alternative lifestyle.
Explain influence of attitude on behavior.	Knowledge of the effect of attitude upon behavior will help patient adapt to personally and culturally acceptable behavior.
Involve patient and partner in psychotherapy if dysfunction affects the relationship.	Communication regarding the dysfunction and plans for intervention is essential to building a healthy, mutually acceptable sexual relationship.
Provide for culturally acceptable sexual enhancement experiences.	Sexual enhancement practices vary from one culture to another and must be compatible with patient's and partner's attitudes and practices.
Discuss acceptable sexual alternatives.	When sexual dysfunction is irreparable, other practices can provide pleasurable alternatives.

▶ NURSING DIAGNOSIS: *Altered Sexuality Patterns*

Related To concern over sexual dysfunction.

Defining Characteristics
- Actual or perceived sexual limitations
- Persistent psychological or biophysical pain
- Performance anxiety
- Absence of sexual satisfaction
- Intense preoccupation with other life activities
- Values conflict
- Fear of alteration in body image

Patient Outcomes
Patient will attain sexual pleasure with partner or upon autostimulation.

Nursing Interventions	Rationales
Take an accurate nursing history.	An accurate history will reveal pertinent biopsychosocial data.
Initiate a one-to-one psychotherapeutic relationship.	A trusting psychotherapeutic relationship is essential for the patient to share diagnosis-related data which may include abuse and violence.
Assess relationship between etiological factor(s) and concern over patient's sexuality.	The etiology is directly related to the intensity of the behavior.
Assess for attitude relative to cultural and religious dictates.	Attitude toward sexuality is determined by religion and culture, which may directly influence a change in sexuality patterns.
Explain influence of attitude on behavior.	Behavior is shaped by attitude. Knowledge of this will give patient insight.
Teach preventative measures.	The seeking of professional help for alterations in sexuality patterns provides an opportunity for teaching illness prevention and contraception.
Teach assertiveness as needed.	An alteration in sexuality patterns may be a signal by a passive partner of abuse or violence. In such a case, assertiveness can become a survival mechanism.
Initiate supportive group therapy.	A support group provides an opportunity for sharing similar conflicts regarding sexuality in a safe, controlled situation.

▶ NURSING DIAGNOSIS: *Spiritual Distress*

Related To preoccupation with sexual dysfunction.

Defining Characteristics

- Questions meaning of own existence
- Alteration in behavior
- Preoccupation
- Anxiety

- Withdrawal
- Anger
- Displacement of anger on partner
- Seeks spiritual guidance
- Sleep pattern alterations

Patient Outcomes

Patient will attain a state of spiritual tranquillity relative to sexual dysfunction.

Nursing Interventions	Rationales
Assess life's philosophy.	Assessment regarding the patient's life philosophy will provide data for planning diagnosis-based intervention.
Assess mental status.	The mental status will determine the type of psychotherapeutic intervention (i.e., if the mental status is too fragile for confrontation).
Assess physical status.	The physical status will determine the level and type of sexual activity that may be possible and will determine alternatives.
Involve patient in supportive individual or group psychotherapy.	Supportive therapy will help build self-image and self-esteem; homogeneous group therapy will show patient that others have similar problems and will reveal alternative coping patterns, thereby helping relieve spiritual distress.
Teach alternative methods of sexual behavior congruent with patient's values and cultural mores.	Alternative coping patterns will serve to substitute for perceived sexual dysfunction, thereby relieving spiritual tension.
Request consultation with clergy if indicated.	Talking to a clergy of one's faith can provide knowledge regarding viable alternative coping mechanisms as well as relieve spiritual distress.

CONTINUITY OF CARE/DISCHARGE PLANNING

- Continue individual or group supportive psychotherapy.
- Refer to sex therapist.
- Refer for appropriate medical intervention if indicated.

BIBLIOGRAPHY

American Psychiatric Association (APA). (1994). *Diagnostic and statistical manual of mental disorders,* (4th ed.). Washington, DC: APA.

Burgess, A. (1990). *Psychiatric nursing in the hospital and the community.* Norwalk, CT: Appleton & Lange.

Fitzpatrick, J. (1991). Taxonomy II: Definitions and development. In R. Carroll-Johnson (Ed.), *Classification of nursing diagnoses. Proceedings of the Ninth Conference of the North American Nursing Diagnosis Association.* Philadelphia, PA: Lippincott.

McConaghy, N. (1993). *Sexual behavior: problems and management.* New York: Plenum.

North American Nursing Diagnosis Association (NANDA). (1992). *NANDA nursing diagnoses: Definitions and classification 1992.* St. Louis, MO: NANDA.

Task Force on *DSM-IV,* American Psychiatric Association (APA). (1993). *DSM-IV draft criteria.* Washington, DC: APA.

Valentin, C. (1992). Personal identity disturbance. In K. Gettrust & P. Brabec (Eds.), *Nursing diagnosis in clinical practice.* Albany, NY: Delmar.

VandeVusse, L. (1992). Spiritual distress. In K. Gettrust & P. Brabec (Eds.), *Nursing diagnosis in clinical practice.* Albany, NY: Delmar.

VandeVusse, L., & Simandl, G. (1992). Sexuality patterns, altered. In K. Gettrust & P. Brabec (Eds.), *Nursing diagnosis in clinical practice.* Albany, NY: Delmar.

Von Best, W. (1992). Sexual dysfunction. In K. Gettrust and P. Brabec (Eds.), *Nursing diagnosis in clinical practice.* Albany, NY: Delmar.

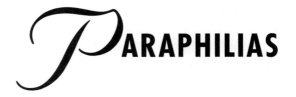

PARAPHILIAS

Marga Simon Coler, EdD, RN, CS, CTN, FAAN

Paraphilias are sexual disorders characterized by intense sexual urges and sexually arousing fantasies deviating from the biological norm. Included in the classification of Paraphilias are Pedophilia, Voyeurism, Exhibitionism, Frotteurism, Transvestic Fetishism, Sexual Masochism, Sexual Sadism, and Fetishism. In cases where fantasies are consensual, this diagnosis does not apply. At times multiple *Diagnostic and Statistical Manual* (DSM) diagnoses occur in patients with this disorder, or there may be several Paraphilias present in one individual.

Paraphilias are prevalent in males, with only an occasional case having been reported in females. Of these, Sexual Masochism, the most widely reported with females, has a 20 : 1 male-female ratio (APA, 1994).

Clinical Clip

The preferred stimulus may be highly specific, having given rise to paraphillic-related services (i.e., prostitutes specializing in bondage or domination) that can be purchased.

ETIOLOGIES

- In general, there is no information about predisposing factors for Paraphilias.
- With Fetishism the object may have had special significance in early childhood.
- Many pedophilics were victims of sexual abuse.
- A common folklore of male transvestites is that they were dressed in girls' clothing as punishment during childhood.

CLINICAL MANIFESTATIONS

- Masochism and Sadism involving self and/or a human partner as well as nonhuman objects, children, or nonconsenting persons
- Sexual arousal from paraphilic fantasies
- Acting upon fantasies periodically during episodes of stress

CLINICAL/DIAGNOSTIC FINDINGS

- The acting on recurrent sexual fantasies and urges to objects that are not part of the normal sexual arousal response patterns

▶ NURSING DIAGNOSIS: *Spiritual Distress*

Related To obsessive thinking about, and compulsive acting out on non-acceptable sexual behavior.

Defining Characteristics

- Obsessional thinking regarding abnormal sexual practices
- Compulsive antisocial behavior regarding abnormal sexual practices
- Frustration at incompleted arousal acts
- Chronic low self-esteem

Patient Outcomes

Patient will be content in using socially acceptable sexual behavior.

Clinical Clip

- Psychotherapy should be conducted by a therapist of the same sex as the patient to enhance communication of a highly sensitive subject.
- Total self-disclosure of incestuous activity is necessary to establish a trusting relationship.

Nursing Interventions	Rationales
Establish a trusting relationship assuring patient of confidentiality.	A trusting relationship is imperative to eliciting a behavioral change.
In individual psychotherapy assess the intensity and lethality of paraphilia.	Thinking patterns influence behavior; restructured thinking may be a first step toward spiritual contentment.

Nursing Interventions	Rationales
Assess the mental status of patient.	The mental status will indicate what type of psychotherapeutic intervention is indicated.
Restructure thinking style of patient.	The aim of psychotherapy is to help the patient adapt to societal norms.
Focus on positive aspects in patient's life.	Paraphiliacs feel overwhelmingly inadequate.
Encourage patient to set small attainable goals.	Small goals will help patient feel a sense of progress.
Teach stress management.	The specific behavior of the individual with paraphilia is frequently brought on by stress.
Teach patient basic communication skills.	Individuals with paraphilia have difficulty in displaying intimacy. They are frequently socially inadequate.

▶ **NURSING DIAGNOSIS:** *High Risk for Violence (Directed at Others)*

Risk Factors
- Stress
- Anxiety
- Fear
- Bizarre imagery

Patient Outcomes
Patient will
- modify paraphiliac urges.
- exercise control over maladaptive behavior.

Nursing Interventions	Rationales
Assess patient for past history of violence.	Past acts of violence are the best predictors in determining at risk for violent behavior.
Conduct a mental status examination with particular emphasis on thought content (i.e., aggressive urges, impulsivity, etc.).	Aggressive thoughts and a high impulsivity level can predict aggressive behavior. Conflicts that fuel rage reactions can be revealed through a thorough mental status

Nursing Interventions	Rationales
	examination combined with psychological testing.
Assess neurological functioning.	Cortical dysfunction has been associated with aggressiveness.
Assess for ego strength.	Assessment of ego functioning will help to determine patient's capacity to benefit from psychotherapeutic intervention.
Initiate systemic desensitization using operant conditioning as needed.	Behavior modification may be useful when patient does not have insight or desire to stop maladaptive behavior.

▶ **NURSING DIAGNOSIS:** *High Risk for Self-Mutilation*

Risk Factors
- Obsessive-compulsive behavior
- Impulsively and compulsively acting out of sexual obsessions
- Masochistic behavior in acting out of sexual fantasy
- External stimuli

Patient Outcomes
Patient will not engage in self-mutilation.

Nursing Interventions	Rationales
Establish a trusting relationship through supportive individual and/or group therapy.	A trusting relationship is essential if patient is to inform therapist or significant other when he or she is ready to act out in a threatening manner.
Assess mental status, including content of obsessional thoughts and previous self-mutilating behavior.	Psychotherapy will be based on preventing self-mutilation.
Consider initiating psychodynamic psychotherapy.	Psychodynamic psychotherapy is employed to gain insight into thought, feeling, and behaviors of patient.

Nursing Interventions	Rationales
Consider initiating behavior modification.	Behavior modification is frequently employed by using operant conditioning to modify fantasies through guided imagery.
Follow up.	Follow-up is imperative as a monitoring device.

CONTINUITY OF CARE/DISCHARGE PLANNING
- Maintain monthly follow-up visits until patient expresses social comfort and demonstrates socially acceptable behavior.
- Monitor thought processes through interaction and psychological testing.
- Refer to paraphiliac support group.
- Refer to social skills training group.

BIBLIOGRAPHY

American Psychiatric Association (APA). (1994). *Diagnostic and statistical manual of mental disorders*, (4th ed.). Washington, DC: APA.

Burgess, A. (1990). *Psychiatric nursing in the hospital and the community.* Norwalk, CT: Appleton & Lange.

Goldman, H. (1988). *General psychiatry.* Norwalk, CT: Appleton & Lange.

McConaghy, N. (1993). *Sexual behavior, problems and management.* New York: Plenum.

North American Nursing Diagnosis Association (NANDA). (1992). *NANDA nursing diagnoses: Definitions and classification 1992.* St. Louis, MO: NANDA.

Task Force on *DSM-IV*, American Psychiatric Association (APA). (1993). *DSM-IV draft criteria.* Washington, DC: APA.

VandeVusse, L. (1992). Spiritual distress. In K. Gettrust & P. Brabec (Eds.), *Nursing diagnosis in clinical practice.* Albany, NY: Delmar.

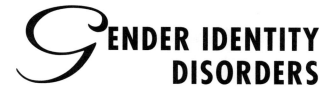

GENDER IDENTITY DISORDERS

Marga Simon Coler, EdD, RN, CS, CTN, FAAN

The classification of Gender Identity Disorders refers to a strong and persistent cross gender identification and a persistent discomfort about one's assigned sex (that which was recorded on the birth certificate). The individual has not only a strong desire to be of the other sex, but may insist that he or she is of that sex and express that gender publicly. Gender identity may be discrete or on a continuum. No recent studies address the prevalence of Gender Identity Disorders. They generally begin in childhood (APA, 1994).

ETIOLOGIES
- Physical characteristics which suggest other than assigned sex
- Separation anxiety
- Non- or weak reinforcement of normative gender role behavior by parents

CLINICAL MANIFESTATIONS
- Stated desire to be other than one's assigned sex
- Frequent passing as other than one's assigned sex
- Desire to be treated as other than one's assigned sex
- Conviction that one has the reactions and feelings as other than one's assigned sex

CLINICAL/DIAGNOSTIC FINDINGS
- There may be a chromosomal or genetic anomaly.
- The patient may have a history of strong role models only of the opposite sex (i.e., a male child being raised in a household of only women).

▶ NURSING DIAGNOSIS: *Altered Role Performance*

Related To a perception of sexual role different than one's assigned sexual role.

Defining Characteristics
- Self-perception of role contrary to one's assigned role
- Conflict between assigned role and one's perception of role
- Stated desire to function in role contrary to one's assigned role
- Wearing attire of sex opposite to one's biological sex
- Performing activities of sex opposite to one's biological sex
- Subjective and/or objective discomfort in the gender role of one's biological sex

Patient Outcomes
Patient will be psychologically and socially at ease with his or her choice of sexual identity.

Nursing Interventions	Rationales
Conduct a complete physical and mental status examination.	Identification of physical and emotional problems helps patient identify realistic goals.
Initiate aversive therapy as needed.	Some success has been demonstrated that associating unpleasant stimuli and responses with pleasures of transsexuality has proved beneficial to those seeking therapeutic intervention.
Initiate therapy to help patient accommodate to his or her chosen gender role without other types of interventions.	Little in the way of psychotherapy or surgery has been found to be helpful.

▶ NURSING DIAGNOSIS: *High Risk for Spiritual Distress*

Risk Factors
- Sexual mores of culture
- Sleep pattern disturbance
- Conflicting thoughts regarding sexual identity
- Increasing marital conflict
- Lack of support system

Patient Outcomes
Patient will
* find support.
* work out conflicts between biological and psychological gender.

Nursing Interventions	Rationales
Help patient find a continuous support person with whom to discuss gender identity conflicts (therapist, clergy).	Generally, psychotherapy has not been found to be therapeutically beneficial. It is therefore imperative that a support system be negotiated.
Initiate supportive group therapy.	Homogeneous groups may be beneficial for finding psychological support for spiritual distress.
Initiate couples' therapy.	Couples may learn to function adaptively with the patient's gender identity conflict.

▶ **NURSING DIAGNOSIS:** *Altered Growth and Development*

Related To increasing awareness of gender identity conflict.

Defining Characteristics
* Difficulty in performing sexual functions of assigned gender
* Difficulty in having sexual feelings of assigned gender
* Considering self to have physical and emotional disability related to preferred gender role

Patient Outcomes
Patient will function contentedly in preferred gender role.

Nursing Interventions	Rationales
Assess physical and psychological growth.	Knowledge of cause and the developmental period of the occurrence of the physical and/or emotional gender role conflict will help in the planning of a therapeutic program.
Initiate values clarification in a supportive environment.	Supportive therapy will help patient define and prioritize values.

Nursing Interventions	Rationales
Help patient be comfortable with his or her gender identity.	The patient will need to adapt to his or her gender identity within the cultural norms of physical and emotional maturation.

▶ NURSING DIAGNOSIS: *Body Image Disturbance*
Related To gender identity conflict.

Defining Characteristics
- Conflict between assigned gender role and one's perceived gender role
- Powerlessness
- Hopelessness
- Verbalization of change in life-style

Patient Outcomes
Patient will perceive self as a healthy human being.

Nursing Interventions	Rationales
Assess physical and psychological growth.	Knowledge of cause and the developmental period of the occurrence of the physical and/or emotional gender role conflict will help in the planning of a therapeutic program.
Initiate values clarification therapy in a supportive environment.	Supportive therapy will help patient define and prioritize values.
Help patient be comfortable with his or her gender identity.	The patient will need to adapt to his or her gender identity within the cultural norms of physical and emotional maturation.

CONTINUITY OF CARE/DISCHARGE PLANNING
- Identify a support system for patient.
- Follow up by telephone monthly to biannually.

BIBLIOGRAPHY

American Psychiatric Association (APA). (1994). *Diagnostic and statistical manual of mental disorders,* (4th ed.). Washington, DC: APA.

Burgess, A. (1990). *Psychiatric nursing in the hospital and the community.* Norwalk, CT: Appleton & Lange.

Eliers, M. (1992). In K. Gettrust & P. Brabec (Eds.), *Nursing diagnosis in clinical practice.* Albany, NY: Delmar.

McConaghy, N. (1993). *Sexual behavior, problems and management.* New York: Plenum.

North American Nursing Diagnosis Association (NANDA). (1992). *NANDA nursing diagnoses: Definitions and classification 1992.* St. Louis, MO: NANDA.

Sheldon, J., & Gollinger, M. (1992). Body image disturbance. In K. Gettrust & P. Brabec (Eds.), *Nursing diagnosis in clinical practice.* Albany, NY: Delmar.

Stuart, G., & Sundeen, S. (1991). *Principles and practice of psychiatric nursing.* St. Louis, MO: Mosby-Year Book.

Task Force on *DSM-IV,* American Psychiatric Association (APA). (1993). *DSM-IV draft criteria.* Washington, DC: APA.

VandeVusse, L. (1992). Spiritual distress. In K. Gettrust & P. Brabec (Eds.), *Nursing diagnosis in clinical practice.* Albany, NY: Delmar.

Eating Disorders

Lenore U. Boles, MS, RN, CS

Characteristically, eating disorders are gross disturbances in eating behaviors. These include Anorexia Nervosa and Bulimia Nervosa, which are related and typically begin in adolescence or early adulthood. There is a third diagnostic category, Eating Disorder Not Otherwise Specified, for eating disorders that do not meet the criteria of Anorexia Nervosa and Bulimia Nervosa. The disorders Pica and Rumination Disorder of Infancy are primarily disorders of young children and probably are not related to the others and will not be discussed here.

The eating disorders are represented by nursing diagnoses in the human response patterns (HRPs) choosing, exchanging, feeling, perceiving, and relating as follows:

HRP	Nursing Diagnosis	Related To
Choosing	Ineffective individual coping	The preoccupation with body image which replaces tasks of appropriate developmental sequences
Exchanging	Altered nutrition: more than body requirements	Food is exchanged or used as a reward or punishment at an unconscious level

HRP	Nursing Diagnosis	Related To
	Altered nutrition: less than body requirements	Food is exchanged or used as a reward or punishment at an unconscious level
Feeling	Anxiety	The use of food and/or alcohol to offset apprehensions of conflicts
	High risk for self-mutilation	The use of food and/or alcohol to offset apprehensions of conflicts
Perceiving	Body image disturbance	Maintaining control when life seems out of control
	Self-esteem disturbance	Maintaining control when life seems out of control
	Powerlessness	Maintaining control when life seems out of control
Relating	Altered family processes	Food is linked to or substituted for relationships

Nursing Interventions	Rationales
Complete a data base including biopsychosocial history.	A complete history is a basis for planning interventions and patient outcomes.
Encourage verbal expression of feelings/conflicts/fears, including those of childhood and self-harm.	Verbal expressions often serve to replace nonproductive eating behaviors as a means of expressing emotional conflict.
Discuss factors that influence eating behaviors.	Adequate nutrition is essential for healthy physical and emotional functioning.
Encourage eating well: three small meals per day and nutritious snacks of fresh fruits/vegetables.	Meal-planning experience is often lacking in young people.
Demonstrate breathing and relaxation exercises.	Relaxation and physical exercises relieve anxiety, painful feelings, and stress.
Plan exercises that will be appropriate.	Patient has knowledge deficit regarding such tools and will

Nursing Interventions	Rationales
	benefit greatly by being able to practice them.
Identify stressors.	Identification of stressors allows for changes in perception and behavior.
Discuss factors that influence perceptions of desirable shape.	Understanding conflicting messages helps to sort them out.
Encourage emphasis on positive physical attributes.	A recognition of positive attributes builds self-esteem.
Work towards acceptance of body.	Acceptance of own body helps build a positive self-image.
Support independent actions and decision making.	Success increases self-esteem.
Give positive feedback when appropriate.	Acceptance encourages positive feelings.
Suggest tools for increasing self-confidence (i.e., positive affirmations).	Independent thinking/actions increase ego strength.
Encourage identification of strengths and weaknesses.	Feedback about strengths and weaknesses promotes self-awareness, which leads to changes.
Model clear communication techniques.	Clear communication facilitates functional relationships.
Demonstrate and acknowledge use of assertive behaviors.	Success encourages further attempts to assert control.
Explore ways of opening family secrets for discussion.	Sharing demonstrates concern, thereby inducing awareness.
Meet with family and patient together.	Through discussions of feelings, families learn new ways of relating to others. Involving family in therapy will allow for reconciliation.
Help to identify appropriate behaviors for family members.	Hurtful behaviors have to be acknowledged and explored before they can be changed.

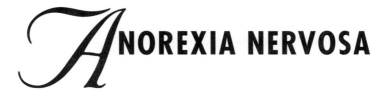

ANOREXIA NERVOSA

Lenore U. Boles, MS, RN, CS

Anorexia Nervosa is a clinical syndrome in which the person has a morbid fear of obesity. It is characterized by the individual's gross distortion of body image, preoccupation with food, and refusal to eat. Manifestations include (1) an intense fear of gaining weight or becoming fat, even though underweight; (2) refusal to maintain body weight, over a minimally normal weight for age and height; (3) failure to make expected weight gain during period of growth, leading to body weight 15% below that expected; (4) disturbance in the perception of one's body weight, size, or shape; (5) undue influence of body weight or shape on self-evaluation or denial of the seriousness of the current low body weight; and, in females, (6) the absence of at least three consecutive menstrual cycles.

The subtypes are (1) Binge Eating/Purging Type, when an individual has recurrent episodes of binge eating during the episode of Anorexia Nervosa, and (2) Restricting Type, when an individual does not engage in recurrent episodes of binge eating during the episode of Anorexia Nervosa.

ETIOLOGIES
- Body image distortion
- Low self-esteem
- Personal vulnerability
- Dysfunctional family of origin
- Feelings of loss of control over one's life
- History of abuse: emotional, physical, sexual, incestuous
- Participation in rigorous athletic programs (particularly team sports)
- Primarily adolescent females

CLINICAL MANIFESTATIONS
- Preoccupation with physical appearance and/or weight and preparation and/or eating of food
- Secretive and/or solitary eating behaviors

- Repeated verbalizations of fears of weight gain
- Use of food for compensation, reward, or reduction of stress
- Prolonged or excessive exercise programs
- Repeated infections
- Fatigue and/or impaired concentration
- Distancing and avoidance behaviors
- In females, lack of development of secondary sexual characteristics and/or cessation of menstrual cycle without other pathology
- Use of cigarettes and/or alcohol to diminish hunger
- Obsession with food
- Organic brain syndrome
- Insomnia
- Depression

CLINICAL/DIAGNOSTIC FINDINGS
- Decrease in pulse and heart rate
- Decrease in blood pressure
- Acrocyanosis
- Heart arrhythmias due to loss of heart muscle
- Compensatory hypothyroidism
- Decrease in body temperature
- Decreased reflexes
- Growth retardation
- Amenorrhea
- Constipation
- Anemia
- Aplastic anemia
- Bone marrow depression
- Flattened facies
- Loss of body fat
- Generalized loss of muscle tissue
- Body weight < 15% of expected norm

▶ NURSING DIAGNOSIS: *Ineffective Individual Coping*

Related To
- Situational crises
- Maturational crises
- Personal vulnerability

Defining Characteristics
- Stated inability to cope or ask for help
- Unable to meet basic needs
- Unable to problem solve
- Changes in social participation
- Self-destructive behaviors

- Changes in communication patterns
- High illness rate
- Increasingly accident prone
- Changes in eating and sleeping patterns
- Physical complaints/symptoms
- Obsessive thinking
- Poor role modeling for dealing with stress
- Internalization of distress: may feel sad, rejected, out of control, frustrated, irritable, tense, directionless, empty inside, angry, hurt, hopeless, lonely, guilty, helpless, and/or powerless

Patient Outcomes
Patient will
- identify and use more productive coping behaviors.
- identify and respond to internal cues for hunger or satiation.
- discuss feelings about self with appropriate supportive significant others.
- identify healthy ways to feel in control of self.

Nursing Interventions	Rationales
Complete a data base, including a biopsychosocial history.	A complete history is a basis for planning interventions and patient outcomes.
Encourage verbal expression of feelings/conflicts.	This would serve to replace non-productive eating behaviors as a means of expressing emotional conflict.
Plan mealtimes to avoid eating alone.	Companionship encourages appropriate eating behaviors.
Demonstrate breathing and relaxation exercises.	Exercise provides an alternative and healthier way to cope with painful feelings and stress.

▶ NURSING DIAGNOSIS: *Altered Nutrition—Less Than Body Requirements*

Related To
- Diminished intake of food in relation to metabolic need
- Psychological factors

Defining Characteristics
- Body weight < 20% of ideal
- Reported inadequate food intake
- Aversion to eating

- Preoccupation with food, especially buying and preparing

Patient Outcomes

Patient will
- increase intake of food.
- identify eating patterns that contribute to undereating.
- gain weight as appropriate.
- decrease physical exercise/activity according to physiological need.

Nursing Interventions	Rationales
Encourage eating well: three small meals per day and nutritious snacks of fresh fruits/vegetables.	Adequate nutrition is essential for healthy physical and emotional functioning; meal-planning experience is often lacking in young people.
Offer nutritional counseling.	Nutritional counseling educates patient regarding needs (food group and caloric distribution).
Plan exercises that will be appropriate.	Conservation or utilization of calories is needed for weight gain.
Structure mealtimes with patient.	Solitary eating encourages unhealthy eating patterns.

▶ NURSING DIAGNOSIS: *Anxiety*

Related To
- Unconscious conflict about essential values/goals of life
- Threat to self-concept
- Situational/maturational crises
- Unmet needs
- Unresolved childhood fears and traumas

Defining Characteristics

- Painful/persistent increased helplessness
- May feel scared, regretful, apprehensive, tense, jittery, inadequate, and/or shaky
- Vague nonspecific fears and concerns
- Sympathetic stimulation, cardiovascular excitation
- Superficial vasoconstriction
- Pupil dilation

- Insomnia
- Poor eye contact
- Trembling/hand tremors
- Facial tension
- Voice quivering
- Focus on "self"
- Increased perspiration
- Narrowing of perceptual field
- Physical and/or emotional withdrawal

Patient Outcomes

Patient will
- examine old fears and beliefs.
- identify some of the factors that induce distress.
- utilize learned behaviors to diminish level of anxiety.

Nursing Interventions	Rationales
Encourage discussion of fears including those of childhood.	Bringing into awareness allows for changes in perception.
Identify stressors.	Identification of stressors allows for changes in thinking and behavior.
Practice stress-reducing techniques.	Relaxation and physical exercises relieve anxiety.

▶ NURSING DIAGNOSIS: *Body Image Disturbance*

Related To
- Perceptual, psychosocial, cultural, and emotional factors
- Mild obesity in adolescence

Defining Characteristics
- Verbalizing negative feelings about body
- Perception of body size/weight not congruent with reality
- Preoccupation with need to become thinner

Patient Outcomes

Patient will
- set realistic goals regarding body size.
- identify cultural/social factors that encourage thinness, especially for women.
- accept positive features about body.

Nursing Interventions	Rationales
Discuss factors that influence perceptions of desirable shape.	Understanding conflicting messages helps to sort them out.
Encourage emphasis on positive physical attributes.	A recognition of positive attributes builds self-esteem.
Work toward acceptance of body.	Acceptance of own body helps build a positive self-image.

▶ NURSING DIAGNOSIS: *Self-Esteem Disturbance*

Related To
- Personal vulnerability
- Mild obesity in adolescence
- Dysfunctional family of origin
- Repeated negative feedback in childhood

Defining Characteristics
- Negative statements about self
- Evaluating self as unable to deal with events
- Rationalizing away/rejecting positive feedback about self
- Denial of problems obvious to others
- Hypersensitivity to slight or criticism
- Body tension
- Giggling when nervous and/or inappropriate to content
- Not in touch with own feelings
- Problem relationship with one or both parents
- Inadequate or poor role models
- Questioning own decisions
- Vacillating over commitments
- Emotionally distant or unavailable
- Repeated relationship difficulties and/or failures
- Seeing self as responsible for relationship problems
- Internalizing distress/stress: may feel empty inside, directionless, sad, angry, anxious, hurt, lonely, guilty, frustrated, ashamed, helpless, worthless, and/or fearful
- Dependent
- Physical symptoms of stress/distress
- History of abuse: physical, emotional, sexual, incestuous
- Allowing self to be manipulated by others
- Unable to accept self
- History of promiscuity
- History of ethyl alcohol (ETOH) and/or drug abuse

Patient Outcomes
Patient will
- develop confidence in own abilities.
- verbalize positive feelings about self.
- make appropriate independent decisions.
- develop and maintain healthy relationships.

Nursing Interventions	Rationales
Support independent actions and decision making.	Success increases self-esteem.
Give positive feedback when appropriate.	Acceptance encourages positive feelings.
Suggest tools for increasing self-confidence (i.e., positive affirmations).	Patient lacks adequate ego strength.
Encourage identification of strengths and weaknesses.	Self-awareness leads to changes.
Model clear communication techniques.	Clear communications facilitate functional relationships.

▶ NURSING DIAGNOSIS: *Powerlessness*

Related To
- Interpersonal interactions
- Emotionally distant and/or rigid, controlling parents

Defining Characteristics
- Expression of having no control or influence over situation and/or outcome
- Reluctance to express feelings
- Inability to please significant other(s)
- Repeated conflict with significant other(s)
- Passive/aggressive acting-out behaviors
- Attention-getting behaviors inappropriate for age/stage
- Social constraints perceived as age/stage inappropriate
- May feel hopeless, helpless, empty inside, directionless, frustrated, and/or depressed
- Fears alienation from significant other(s)

Patient Outcomes
Patient will
- express feelings and conflicts in appropriate ways.
- exercise control over own life appropriate to age and stage.
- use assertive behaviors rather than passive/aggressive ones.

Nursing Interventions	Rationales
Encourage verbal expression of feelings and conflicts.	Adults use verbal language to convey messages.
Assist with specific plans in one or two areas of life that will give quick results.	Success encourages further attempts to assert control.
Demonstrate and acknowledge use of assertive behaviors.	Modeling provides guidelines for growth.

▶ NURSING DIAGNOSIS: *Altered Family Processes*

Related To
• Dysfunctional family
• Substance abuse
• Incest

Defining Characteristics
• Family system unable to meet emotional needs of members
• Inability to express/accept feelings of members
• Inability to meet security needs of members
• Inability to relate to each other for mutual growth and maturation
• Inability to receive/accept help appropriately
• Rigidity in function and roles
• Does not demonstrate respect for individuality and autonomy of its members
• Failure to send/receive clear messages
• Rigidity of positions (taken/guarded)
• Inappropriate boundary crossing

Patient Outcomes
Patient will
• express/accept own feelings.
• confront unacceptable behavior within the family system.
• discuss needs/expectations with family members.
• feel safe when with family members.

Nursing Interventions	Rationales
Encourage discussion of feelings.	Through discussions of feelings family members learn a new way of relating to others.

Nursing Interventions	Rationales
Explore ways of opening family secrets for discussion.	Hurtful behaviors have to be acknowledged and explored before they can be changed.
Help to identify appropriate behaviors for family members.	Positive role modeling encourages identification with new behaviors.

CONTINUITY OF CARE/DISCHARGE PLANNING
- Encourage ongoing family, individual, and/or group psychotherapy (i.e., long-term, intensive, insight therapy; short-term intensive therapy).
- Arrange for continued medical supervision.
- Monitor for necessity for pharmacological intervention (i.e., antidepressant medication).
- Advise that rehospitalization may be necessary if weight falls below a physiologically safe level.
- Provide short-term antianxiety medications if patient is unable to complete activities of daily living.

BIBLIOGRAPHY

American Psychiatric Association (APA). (1994). *Diagnostic and statistical manual of mental disorders,* (4th ed.). Washington, DC: APA.

Dardis, P., & Hofland, S. (1990). Anorexia nervosa. *Journal of Child and Adolescent Psychiatry and Mental Health Nursing, 3*(3), 85–90.

Fitzpatrick, J. (1991). Taxonomy II: Definitions and development. In R. Carroll-Johnson (Ed.), *Classification of nursing diagnoses. Proceedings of the Ninth Conference of the North American Nursing Diagnosis Association.* Philadelphia, PA: Lippincott.

Forisha, B., Grothaus, K., & Luscombe, R. (1990). Dinner conversation. *Journal of Psychosocial Nursing, 28*(11), 12–16.

Kiecolt-Glaser, J., & Dixon, K. (1984). Postadolescent onset male anorexia. *Journal of Psychosocial Nursing, 22*(1), 11–20.

Lewis, S., & Collier, I. (1992). *Medical surgical nursing.* St. Louis, MO: Mosby-Year Book.

North American Nursing Diagnosis Association (NANDA). (1992). *NANDA nursing diagnoses: Definitions and classification 1992.* St. Louis, MO: NANDA.

Staples, N., & Schwartz, M. (1990). Anorexia nervosa support group: Providing transitional support. *Journal of Psychosocial Nursing, 28*(2), 6–10.

Task Force on *DSM-IV*, American Psychiatric Association (APA). (1991). *DSM-IV options book: Work in progress.* Washington, DC: APA.

Townsend, M. (1988). *Nursing diagnoses in psychiatric nursing.* Philadelphia, PA: Davis.

Whitley, G. (1989). Anxiety. *Journal of Psychosocial Nursing, 27*(10), 7–12.

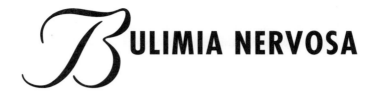

BULIMIA NERVOSA

Lenore U. Boles, MS, RN, CS

Bulimia Nervosa is commonly called the "Binge-and-Purge Syndrome" and is characterized by extreme overeating followed by self-induced vomiting and abuse of laxatives and diuretics. Self-evaluation is radically influenced by body shape and weight. The diagnosis is not made if the binge eating and subsequent behaviors have not occurred at least twice per week for three months. Bulimia does not occur only during episodes of Anorexia Nervosa. There are two subtypes: (1) Purging Type, in which an individual regularly engages in the use of laxatives or diuretics or in self-induced vomiting, and (2) Nonpurging Type, where the individual does not regularly engage in purging but reverts to strict dieting, fasting, or vigorous exercise. (APA, 1994, pp. 545–550)

ETIOLOGIES
- Body image distortion
- Low self-esteem
- Personal vulnerability
- Dysfunctional family of origin
- Feelings of loss of control over one's life
- Incest
- Sexual, emotional, or physical abuse in childhood
- Participation in rigorous athletic programs (particularly team sports)
- In females, cessation of menstrual cycle without other pathology
- Adolescence especially females, with growing incidence in males (usually those engaged in highly competitive high school sports)
- Use of cigarettes and/or alcohol to diminish hunger and/or to facilitate vomiting

CLINICAL MANIFESTATIONS
- Recurrent episodes of binge eating which may be considerably more than most people would eat

- A sense of lack of control over eating during the episode which occurs in a discrete period of time
- A recurrent maladaptive compensatory behavior, such as
  −self-induced vomiting
  −abuse of laxatives and/or diuretics
  −excessive exercise to prevent weight gain
- Two binge-eating episodes a week for at least 3 months
- Secretive or solitary eating behaviors
- Flattened facies
- Obsession with food
- Insomnia or excessive sleeping
- Poor concentration
- Depression

CLINICAL/DIAGNOSTIC FINDINGS

- Blood volume depletion
- Dehydration
- Decrease in blood pressure/heart rate
- Electrolyte imbalance
- Cardiomyopathy and/or myocarditis
- Cardiac arrhythmias
- Parotid and salivary gland enlargement
- Compensatory hypothyroidism
- Decreased body temperature
- Decreased reflexes
- Reflex hypofunctioning of the bowel and constipation
- Hemorrhoids and rectal discomfort
- Occult bleeding
- Steatorrhea
- Esophageal tears and/or gastric ruptures
- Anemia
- Dental erosion and/or oral cavity trauma
- Halitosis
- Edema
- Generalized loss of muscle tissue
- Sudden death

▶ NURSING DIAGNOSIS: *Ineffective Individual Coping*

Related To
- Situational crises
- Maturational crises
- Personal vulnerability

Defining Characteristics
- Stated inability to cope or ask for help
- Inability to meet basic needs
- Inability to problem solve
- Changes in social participation
- Self-destructive behaviors
- Changes in communication patterns
- High illness rate

- Increasingly accident prone
- Changes in eating and sleeping patterns
- Physical complaints/symptoms
- Obsessive thinking
- Poor role models for dealing with stress
- Internalization of distress: may feel sad, rejected, out of control, frustrated, irritable, tense, directionless, empty inside, angry, hurt, hopeless, lonely, guilty, and/or helpless

Patient Outcomes
Patient will
- identify and use more productive coping behaviors.
- identify and respond to internal cues for hunger or satiation.
- discuss feelings about self with appropriate supportive significant others.
- identify healthy ways to feel in control of self.

Nursing Interventions	Rationales
Complete a data base which includes a biopsychosocial history.	A thorough history is the basis for planning interventions and patient outcomes.
Encourage verbal expression of feelings/conflicts.	Verbal communication serves to replace nonproductive eating behaviors as a means of expression of emotional conflict.
Plan mealtimes to avoid eating alone.	Companionship encourages appropriate eating behaviors.

▶ **NURSING DIAGNOSIS:** *Altered Nutrition—More Than Body Requirements*

Related To
- Excessive intake of food in relation to metabolic need
- Psychological factors

Defining Characteristics
- Eating in response to internal cues other than hunger (i.e., anxiety, loneliness)
- Reported or observed dysfunctional eating pattern

Patient Outcomes
Patient will
- decrease intake of food.

- identify eating patterns that contribute to overeating.
- maintain weight as appropriate.
- increase physical exercise/activity according to physiological need.

Nursing Interventions	Rationales
Encourage eating well (three small meals per day, nutritious snacks of fresh fruits/vegetables).	Adequate nutrition is essential for healthy physical and emotional functioning; meal-planning experience is often lacking in young people.
Provide nutritional counseling.	Nutritional counseling will provide knowledge regarding nutritional needs (food group and caloric distribution).
Structure mealtimes with patient.	Solitary eating encourages unhealthy eating patterns.
Plan appropriate exercises.	Conservation or utilization of calories is needed for weight maintenance.

▶ NURSING DIAGNOSIS: *Anxiety*

Related To
- Unconscious conflict about essential values/goals of life
- Threat to self-concept
- Situational/maturational crises
- Unmet needs
- Unresolved childhood fears and traumas

Defining Characteristics
- Painful/persistent increased helplessness
- May feel nonspecific, vague fear, regretful, jittery, inadequate, restless, and/or uncertain
- Sympathetic stimulation (cardiovascular excitation, superficial vasoconstriction, pupil dilation)
- Insomnia
- Hand tremors, voice quivering, poor eye contact, facial tension
- Diaphoresis
- Narrowing of perceptual field
- Withdrawal (physical and/or emotional)

Patient Outcomes

Patient will

- examine old fears and beliefs.
- identify some of the factors that induce distress.
- utilize learned behaviors to diminish level of anxiety.

Nursing Interventions	Rationales
Encourage discussion of fears, including those of childhood.	Bringing fears into awareness allows for changes in perception.
Identify stressors.	Identifying and confronting stressors allows for changes.
Practice stress-reducing techniques.	Relaxation and physical exercises relieve anxiety.

▶ NURSING DIAGNOSIS: *High Risk for Self-Mutilation*

Risk Factors

- History of self-injury
- History of physical, emotional, or sexual abuse in adolescents or young adults (especially in females)
- Parental emotional deprivation
- Dysfunctional family of origin

Patient Outcomes

Patient will

- express feelings verbally before acting on them.
- examine old fears and beliefs.
- work through feelings related to family.
- accept family as they are.

Nursing Interventions	Rationales
Share with patient when it appears tension is building.	Sharing demonstrates concern, thereby inducing awareness.
Encourage sharing of feelings and thoughts, especially self-destructive ones.	Verbal expression is healthy and permits validation of thoughts and feelings.
Meet with family and patient together.	Involving family in therapy will allow for reconciliation.

▶ NURSING DIAGNOSIS: *Body Image Disturbance*

Related To perceptual, psychosocial, cultural, and emotional factors.

Defining Characteristics
- Verbalizing negative feelings about body
- Perception of body size/weight incongruent with reality
- Preoccupation with need to become thinner

Patient Outcomes
Patient will
- set realistic goals regarding body size.
- identify cultural/social factors that encourage thinness, especially for women.
- accept positive features about body.

Nursing Interventions	Rationales
Discuss factors that influence perceptions of desirable shape.	Understanding conflicting messages helps to sort them out.
Encourage emphasis on positive physical attributes.	Recognizing positive physical attributes will lead to acceptance of body.

▶ NURSING DIAGNOSIS: *Self-Esteem Disturbance*

Related To
- Personal vulnerability
- Dysfunctional family of origin
- Repeated negative feedback in childhood
- Mild obesity in adolescence

Defining Characteristics
- Negative statements about self
- Rationalizing away/rejecting positive feedback about self
- Hypersensitivity to slight or criticism
- Questioning own decisions
- Out of touch with feelings
- Problem relationship with one or both parents
- Inadequate or poor role models
- Vacillating over commitments
- Emotionally distant or unavailable
- Repeated relationship difficulties and/or failures
- Seeing self as responsible for relationship problems

- Internalizing distress/stress: may feel empty inside, directionless, angry, anxious, hurt, lonely, guilty, frustrated, ashamed, helpless, worthless, fearful, and/or sad
- Dependent
- History of abuse: physical, emotional, sexual, incestuous
- Allowing self to be manipulated by others
- Inability to accept self
- History of promiscuity and ethyl alcohol (ETOH) and/or drug abuse
- Verbalizing lack of self-confidence

Patient Outcomes

Patient will
- develop confidence in own abilities.
- verbalize positive feelings about self.
- make appropriate independent decisions.
- develop and maintain healthy relationships.

Nursing Interventions	Rationales
Support independent actions and decision making.	Success increases self-esteem.
Give positive feedback when appropriate.	Acceptance encourages positive feelings.
Suggest tools for increasing self-confidence (i.e., positive affirmations).	Patient has knowledge deficit regarding such tools and will benefit greatly by being able to practice them.
Encourage identification of strengths and weaknesses.	Self-awareness leads to changes.
Model clear communication techniques.	Clear communications will enhance interpersonal relationships.

▶ NURSING DIAGNOSIS: *Powerlessness*

Related To
- Maladaptive interpersonal interactions
- Emotionally distant and/or rigid controlling parents

Defining Characteristics
- Expression of having no control or influence over situation and/or outcome
- Reluctance to express feelings
- Inability to please significant other(s)

- Repeated conflict with significant other(s)
- Passive/aggressive acting-out behaviors (specify)
- Attention-getting behaviors inappropriate for age/stage
- Social constraints perceived as age/stage inappropriate
- May feel hopeless, helpless, empty inside, adrift, directionless, frustrated, and/or depressed
- Fearing alienation from significant other(s)

Patient Outcomes
Patient will
- express feelings and conflicts in appropriate ways.
- exercise control over own life appropriate to age and stage.
- use assertive behaviors rather than passive/aggressive ones.

Nursing Interventions	Rationales
Encourage verbal expression of feelings and conflicts.	Adults use verbal language to convey messages.
Assist with specific plans in one or two areas of life that will give quick results.	Success encourages further attempts to assert control.
Demonstrate and acknowledge use of assertive behaviors.	Modeling and confirmation provide guidelines for growth.

▶ NURSING DIAGNOSIS: *Altered Family Processes*
Related To
- Dysfunctional family
- Substance abuse
- Incest

Defining Characteristics
- Family system unable to meet emotional needs of members
- Inability to express/accept feelings of members
- Inability to meet security needs of members
- Inability to relate to each other for mutual growth and maturation
- Inability to receive/accept help appropriately
- Rigidity in functions, positions, and roles
- Family does not demonstrate respect for individuality and autonomy of its members
- Failure to send/receive clear messages
- Inappropriate boundary crossing

Patient Outcomes
Patient will
- express/accept own feelings.
- confront unacceptable behavior within the family system.
- discuss needs/expectations with family members.
- feel safe when with family members.

Nursing Interventions	Rationales
Encourage discussion of feelings.	Discussion of feelings may be a new way of relating to others.
Explore ways of discussing family secrets.	Hurtful behaviors have to be acknowledged and explored before they can be changed.
Help to identify appropriate behaviors for family members.	Positive role models will encourage identification with new behaviors.

CONTINUITY OF CARE/DISCHARGE PLANNING
- Provide for ongoing family therapy in conjunction with individual and/or group therapy.
- Arrange/encourage continued medical supervision.
- Evaluate for hospitalization as needed.
- Refer for supervised physical exercise and/or activity program.
- Evaluate for psychopharmacological intervention (i.e., short-term antianxiety, antidepressant, and anticonvulsant medications).
- Initiate a suicide contract prn.

BIBLIOGRAPHY

American Psychiatric Association (APA). (1994). *Diagnostic and statistical manual of mental disorders* (4th ed.). Washington, DC: APA.

Hofland, S., & Dardis, P. (1992). Bulimia nervosa. *Journal of Psychosocial Nursing, 30*(2), 23–27.

Kopeski, L. (1989). Diabetes and bulimia: A deadly duo. *American Journal of Nursing, 89*(4), 483–485.

Laraia, M., & Stuart, G. (1990). Bulimia. *Journal of Child and Adolescent Psychiatry and Mental Health Nursing, 3*(3), 91–97.

Lewis, S., & Collier, I. (1992). *Medical surgical nursing.* St. Louis, MO: Mosby Year-Book.

North American Nursing Diagnosis Association (NANDA). (1992). *NANDA nursing diagnoses: Definitions and classification 1992.* St. Louis, MO: NANDA.

Task Force on *DSM-IV*, American Psychiatric Association (APA). (1991). *DSM-IV options book: Work in progress.* Washington, DC: APA.

Townsend, M. (1988). *Nursing diagnoses in psychiatric nursing.* Philadelphia, PA: Davis.

$\mathscr{B}$INGE EATING DISORDER

Lenore U. Boles, MS, RN, CS

Binge Eating Disorder refers to recurrent episodes of eating excessively large quantities of food, without purging, at any one time. The episode is characterized by eating an amount of food that is larger than most people would eat in a similar, discrete period of time. There is also a sense of lack of control over eating during the episode. Binge Eating does not occur exclusively during the course of Bulimia Nervosa, and the individual does not abuse medication in an attempt to avoid weight gain. Binge Eating occurs, on average, at least twice a week for a 6-month period and causes marked distress.

ETIOLOGIES
- Body image distortion
- Low self-esteem
- Personal vulnerability
- Dysfunctional family of origin
- Feelings of loss of control over one's life
- Incest
- Sexual, emotional, or physical abuse in childhood

CLINICAL MANIFESTATIONS
At least three of the following behavioral indicators of loss of control are present during most binge episodes:
- obsession with food
- eating much more rapidly than usual
- eating until feeling uncomfortably full
- eating large amounts of food when not feeling physically hungry and/or with no planned mealtimes
- eating alone because of embarrassment over quantity
- feeling disgusted with oneself, depressed, or guilty after overeating
- insomnia or increased sleep, drowsiness
- impaired concentration

CLINICAL/DIAGNOSTIC FINDINGS
- Cardiovascular and respiratory problems: dyspnea on exertion, orthopnea, paroxysmal nocturnal dyspnea, polycythemia secondary to low oxygenation of arterial blood with resulting occlusion of vessels and clotting abnormalities, increased red blood cell count and blood volume, hypertrophy of the heart, especially of the left ventricle, coronary heart disease, cyanosis, edema
- Reduced vital capacity
- Increase in pulse/heart rate and blood pressure
- Diabetes mellitus
- Menstrual irregularities
- Infertility
- Endometrial cancer
- Compensatory hypothyroidism
- Gallstone formation
- Fatty liver infiltration
- Raised cholesterol and triglyceride levels
- Constipation
- Epigastric distress
- Depression
- Generalized loss of muscle tone/slowed reflexes
- Weight gain

▶ NURSING DIAGNOSIS: *Ineffective Individual Coping*

Related To
- Situational crises
- Maturational crises
- Personal vulnerability

Defining Characteristics
- Stated inability to cope or ask for help
- Inability to problem solve
- Changes in social participation
- Self-destructive behaviors
- Changes in communication patterns
- High illness rate
- Increasingly accident prone
- Changes in eating and sleeping patterns
- Physical complaints/symptoms
- Obsessive thinking
- Poor role modeling for dealing with stress
- Internalization of distress: may feel sad, rejected, out of control, frustrated, irritable, tense, without direction, empty inside, anger, hurt, hopeless, lonely, guilty, helpless, and/or powerless

Patient Outcomes
Patient will
* identify and use more productive coping behaviors.
* identify and respond to internal cues for hunger or satiation.
* discuss feelings about self with appropriate supportive significant others.
* identify healthy ways to feel in control of self.

Nursing Interventions	Rationales
Complete a data base which includes a biopsychosocial history.	A comprehensive history is the basis for planning interventions and patient outcomes.
Encourage verbal expression of feelings/conflicts.	Verbalization might serve to replace nonproductive eating behaviors as means of expression of emotional conflict.
Plan mealtimes to avoid eating alone.	Companionship encourages appropriate eating behaviors.

▶ NURSING DIAGNOSIS: *Altered Nutrition—More Than Body Requirements*

Related To excessive intake of food in relation to metabolic need due to psychological factors.

Defining Characteristics
* Eating in response to internal cues other than hunger (i.e., anxiety, loneliness)
* Reported or observed dysfunctional eating pattern

Patient Outcomes
Patient will
* decrease intake of food.
* identify eating patterns that contribute to overeating.
* maintain weight as appropriate.
* increase physical exercise/activity according to physiological need.

Nursing Interventions	Rationales
Encourage eating well (three small meals a day and nutritious snacks of fresh fruits/vegetables).	Adequate nutrition is essential for healthy physical and emotional functioning.

Nursing Interventions	Rationales
Offer nutritional counseling.	Education regarding nutritional needs is essential (food groups and caloric distribution).
Plan appropriate exercises.	Proper utilization of calories is needed for weight loss.
Structure mealtimes with patient.	Solitary eating encourages unhealthy eating patterns.

▶ NURSING DIAGNOSIS: *Anxiety*

Related To
- Unconscious conflict about essential values/goals of life
- Threat to self-concept
- Situational/maturational crises
- Unmet needs
- Unresolved childhood fears and traumas

Defining Characteristics
- Painful/persistent increased helplessness
- May feel uncertain, scared, regretful, tense, apprehensive, restless, and/or inadequate
- May have vague, nonspecific fears and concerns
- Sympathetic stimulation: cardiovascular excitation, superficial vasoconstriction, pupil dilation
- Insomnia
- Poor eye contact
- Tremors, facial tension
- Focus on "self"
- Diaphoresis
- Narrowing of perceptual field
- Physical and/or emotional withdrawal

Patient Outcomes
Patient will
- examine old fears and beliefs.
- identify some of the factors that induce distress.
- utilize learned behaviors to diminish level of anxiety.

Nursing Interventions	Rationales
Encourage discussion of fears (including those of childhood).	Bringing fears into awareness allows for changes in perception.
Identify stressors.	Identification of stressors allows for changes.
Practice stress-reducing techniques.	Relaxation and physical exercises relieve anxiety.

▶ NURSING DIAGNOSIS: *Body Image Disturbance*

Related To perceptual, psychosocial, cultural, and emotional factors.

Defining Characteristics
• Verbalizing negative feelings about body

Patient Outcomes
Patient will
• set realistic goals regarding eating behaviors.
• accept positive features about self, including body.

Nursing Interventions	Rationales
Discuss factors that influence eating behaviors.	Understanding conflicting messages helps to sort them out.
Encourage emphasis on positive physical attributes.	Recognition of positive attributes is a first step toward acceptance of self.

▶ NURSING DIAGNOSIS: *Self-Esteem Disturbance*

Related To
• Personal vulnerability
• Dysfunctional family of origin
• Repeated negative feedback in childhood

Defining Characteristics
• Negative statements about self
• Rationalizing away/rejecting positive feedback about self
• Hypersensitivity to slight or criticism
• Questioning own decisions

- Not being in touch with own feelings
- Problem relationship with one or both parents
- Inadequate or poor role models
- Vacillating over commitments
- Emotionally distant or unavailable
- Repeated relationship difficulties and/or failures
- Seeing self as responsible for relationship problems
- Internalized distress/stress: may feel empty inside, directionless, sad, angry, anxious, hurt, lonely, frustrated, ashamed, helpless, worthless, and/or fearful
- Dependent
- Physical symptoms of stress/distress
- History of abuse: physical, emotional, sexual
- Allowing self to be manipulated by others
- Unable to accept self
- History of promiscuity and ethyl alcohol (ETOH) and/or drug abuse
- Verbalizing lack of self-confidence

Patient Outcomes

Patient will
- develop confidence in own abilities.
- verbalize positive feelings about self.
- make appropriate independent decisions.
- develop and maintain healthy relationships.

Nursing Interventions	Rationales
Support independent actions and decision making.	Success increases self-esteem.
Give positive feedback when appropriate.	Acceptance encourages positive feelings.
Suggest tools for increasing self-confidence (i.e., positive affirmations).	Self-confidence helps promote self-esteem.
Encourage identification of strengths and weaknesses.	Self-awareness leads to changes.
Model clear communication techniques.	Clear communications facilitate making functional relationships.

▶ NURSING DIAGNOSIS: *Powerlessness*

Related To
- Negative interpersonal interactions
- Emotionally distant and/or rigid, controlling parents

Defining Characteristics
- Expression of having no control or influence over situation and/or outcome
- Reluctance to express feelings
- Inability to please significant other(s)
- Repeated conflict with significant other(s)
- Passive/aggressive acting-out behaviors
- Attention-getting behaviors inappropriate for age/stage
- May feel hopeless, helpless, empty inside, adrift, directionless, frustrated, and/or depressed

Patient Outcomes
Patient will
- express feelings and conflicts in appropriate ways.
- exercise control over own eating behaviors.
- use assertive behaviors rather than passive/aggressive ones.

Nursing Interventions	Rationales
Encourage verbal expression of feelings and conflicts.	Adults use verbal language to convey messages.
Assist with specific plans to control eating that give quick results.	Success encourages further attempts to assert control.
Demonstrate and acknowledge use of assertive behaviors.	Modeling and confirmation provide guidelines for growth.

CONTINUITY OF CARE/DISCHARGE PLANNING
- Arrange for individual, family, and/or group psychotherapy.
- Encourage behavioral therapy as needed.
- Arrange for continuous medical supervision.
- Evaluate for psychopharmacological intervention (i.e., antidepressant and/or antianxiety medications as needed).
- Encourage attendance at support groups (i.e., Overeaters Anonymous).
- Encourage participation in relaxation exercises, physical exercise, and activity programs.

BIBLIOGRAPHY

American Psychiatric Association (APA). (1994). *Diagnostic and statistical manual of mental disorders* (4th ed.). Washington, DC: APA.

Kopeski, L. (1989). Diabetes and bulimia: A deadly duo. *American Journal of Nursing, 89*(4), 483–485.

Lewis, S., & Collier, I. (1992). *Medical surgical nursing.* St. Louis, MO: Mosby-Year Book.

North American Nursing Diagnosis Association (NANDA). (1992). *NANDA nursing diagnoses: Definitions and classification 1992.* St. Louis, MO: NANDA.

Task Force on *DSM-IV,* American Psychiatric Association (APA). (1991). *DSM-IV options book: Work in progress.* Washington, DC: APA.

Townsend, M. (1988). *Nursing diagnoses in psychiatric nursing.* Philadelphia, PA: Davis.

Whitley, G. (1989). Anxiety. *Journal of Psychosocial Nursing, 27*(10), 7–12.

Adjustment Disorders

Helene M. Vartelas, MSN, RN, CS

In the *Diagnostic and Statistical Manual of Mental Disorders*, (4th ed.), the following disorders fall within this category:

- Adjustment Disorder with Depressed Mood (major symptoms include a depressed mood, tearfulness, and feelings of hopelessness)
- Adjustment Disorder with Anxiety (major symptoms are nervousness, worry, and jitteriness)
- Adjustment Disorder with Mixed Anxiety and Depressed Mood (major symptoms show a combination of anxiety and depression)
- Adjustment Disorder with Disturbance of Conduct (major symptoms include violations of the rights of others, societal norms, and rules)
- Adjustment Disorder with Mixed Disturbance of Emotions and Conduct (major symptoms include emotional symptoms and conduct disturbances)
- Adjustment Disorder Unspecified (other extreme reactions to psychosocial stressors such as social withdrawal or inhibited academic responses that are not able to be classified elsewhere).

Adjustment Disorders are caused by a maladaptive reaction to an identifiable psychosocial stressor or stressors that is indicated by one or more of the following:

- impairment in occupational (or school) functioning, usual social activities, and relationships with others
- symptoms that are excessive that would be expected in terms of a normal reaction to stress

The stressor(s) must have had to occur within 3 months of the onset of symptoms but have not persisted for longer than 6 months. This disorder is not a single instance of an overreaction to stress or an exacerbation of another preexisting mental disorder. Stressors may be single (e.g., psychological reaction to a physical illness) or multiple (e.g., foreclosure, loss of relationships, moving) and can occur to an individual person, a family, or a community (e.g., natural disaster).

Adjustment Disorders are represented by nursing diagnoses in the human response patterns (HRPs) choosing, feeling, perceiving, and relating as follows:

HRP	Nursing Diagnosis	Related To
Choosing	Ineffective individual coping	Situational or developmental crises
Feeling	Anxiety	Maladaptive reaction to identifiable stressors
Perceiving	Self-esteem disturbance	Inadequate support systems
Relating	Impaired social interaction	Inadequate support systems

Nursing Interventions

Initiate individual psychotherapy as indicated. This may be in the form of:

1. Insight-oriented psychotherapy which focuses on insight into the dynamics of the patient's thoughts, feeling, behaviors, and relationships.
2. Supportive psychotherapy to restore or strengthen defenses and integrating capacities that may have become dysfunctional.
3. Brief dynamic psychotherapy [i.e., brief psychotherapy (Travistock-Malan); time-limited psychotherapy (Mann);

Rationales

Individual personal meaning of the stressor(s) and its association with earlier life traumas are explored and dealt with. Patients can often emerge with a healthier personality structure than was previously experienced.

1. Insight-oriented therapy assists the patient in gaining insight into the dynamics of thoughts, feelings, behaviors, and relationships.
2. Support is offered by the therapist during the period of crisis or temporary decompensation. Dependency needs are gratified

Nursing Interventions	Rationales
short-term anxiety-provoking psychotherapy (Weissman-Klerman); crisis intervention (Lindermann)].	and the patient develops independence. 3. Brief psychotherapy helps the motivated patient understand psychological concepts and interpretations, toward a goal of resolution of underlying conflicts related to a patient's current situation or problem.
Recommend participation in g roup psychotherapy as needed.	The group context assists the members of the group in exploring the personal meaning of the stressor(s) and provides valuable feedback on coping behaviors.

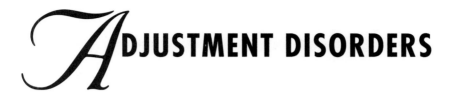

ADJUSTMENT DISORDERS

Helene M. Vartelas, MSN, RN, CS

Adjustment Disorders are not a single instance of an overreaction to stress or an exacerbation of another preexisting mental disorder. The severity of the disorders is often not predictable from stressor intensity. Adjustment Disorders may affect an individual, a family, or a community. Remission generally occurs after cessation of the stressor(s).

ETIOLOGIES
- A maladaptive reaction to an identifiable psychosocial stressor or stressors
- Stressors may be single (e.g., psychological reaction to a physical illness) or multiple (e.g., foreclosure, loss of relationships, moving) and can occur to an individual person, a family, or a community (e.g., natural disaster).

CLINICAL MANIFESTATIONS
- Impairment in occupational (or school) functioning
- Impairment in usual social activities
- Impairment in relationships with others
- Symptoms excessive to what would be expected in terms of a normal reaction to stress
- Symptoms that occur within 3 months after the stressor(s) but have not persisted for longer than 6 months

CLINICAL/DIAGNOSTIC FINDINGS
(None)

▶ NURSING DIAGNOSIS: *Ineffective Individual Coping*
Related To
- Situational and/or developmental crises

- Maladaptive reaction to an identifiable stressor
- Inadequate support systems

Defining Characteristics

- Anxiety
- Depressed mood
- Impaired level of functioning in terms of social roles
- Impaired problem-solving abilities

- Somatic complaints
- Social withdrawal and/or dependency
- Sleep disturbance

Patient Outcomes

Patient will effectively cope with stressors by end of treatment.

Nursing Interventions	Rationales
Assess level of depression and suicide potential; provide a safe environment.	Depressed mood and ineffective coping mechanisms may lead to a potential for suicide. Maintenance of patient safety is a top priority.
Assess level of anxiety.	Anxious mood may lead to diminished problem-solving abilities and diminished abilities to use alternative coping mechanisms.
Provide supportive staff relationships and encourage exploration of positive, effective coping mechanisms.	Trust, the basic building block of the nurse-patient relationship, needs to be developed between nurse and patient so that the patient can begin, with the assistance of the nurse, to not only ventilate the causes of the anxiety but also explore more positive coping mechanisms.
Provide opportunities for the utilization of new positive coping mechanisms through such modalities as role play, interpersonally oriented group therapy, family/significant other therapy sessions, individual counseling/therapy sessions, and daily living situations in the therapeutic milieu.	As the patient begins to feel better, he or she will be able to explore with the nurse current stressors and the ways in which he or she deals with stress. The patient can then broaden repertoire of positive coping mechanisms.

▶ NURSING DIAGNOSIS: *Anxiety*

Related To
- Maladaptive reaction to an identifiable stressor
- Situational and/or developmental crises
- Inadequate support systems

Defining Characteristics
- Anxious mood
- Somatic complaints such as hyperventilation, palpitations, sweating, headaches, or other nonspecific complaints
- Sleep pattern disturbances
- Appetite disturbances
- Loss of libido

Patient Outcomes
Patient will not exhibit signs or symptoms of anxiety by the end of treatment.

Nursing Interventions	Rationales
Assess level of anxiety; provide supportive nurse-patient relationship and opportunities for ventilation regarding feelings of anxiety and their etiology. Provide opportunities for patient to learn to master feelings through regular counseling/therapy sessions; daily journal keeping; development of appropriate release activities such as physical exercise, yoga, relaxation training, meditation, art work, volunteer work, etc.	A supportive nurse-patient relationship will assist the patient in exploring the root causes of his or her anxieties, and once this is done, the patient will have the strength and courage to learn to master these feelings.
Assess appetite and weight loss/gain; assist patient in meal planning and nutritional counseling.	Appetite disturbance can lead to making the patient feel worse and also negatively alter his or her self-concept. Nutritional counseling and assistance with meal planning, often including vitamin supplementation, is necessary to assist the patient in regaining a state of wellness.

Nursing Interventions	Rationales
Assess sleep patterns and assist the patient in reestablishing his or her normal sleep pattern.	Sleep pattern disturbances such as hyposomnia, difficulty falling asleep, midnight awakening and early morning awakening impact negatively on one's overall wellness and need to be attended to in order to assist the patient in regaining an overall state of wellness.

▶ NURSING DIAGNOSIS: *Self-Esteem Disturbance*

Related To
- Maladaptive reaction to an identifiable stressor
- Situational and/or developmental crisis
- Inadequate support systems

Defining Characteristics
- Lowered sense of self-esteem
- Self-deprecating comments
- Feelings of lowered self-worth
- Depressed mood

Patient Outcomes
Patient will demonstrate a positive self-concept by the end of treatment.

Nursing Interventions	Rationales
Assess level of depression and suicide potential; provide for a safe environment.	The level of depression and potential for suicide must be monitored to ensure patient safety. A safe environment encourages the patient to verbalize feelings and also to know that the feelings can be contained and constructively worked with.
Assist the patient in seeking out and participating in ego-enhancing activities.	Self-esteem is enhanced by recognizing the positive aspects of one's personality and life and experiencing these through ego-enhancing activities. This results in growth toward a more positive sense of self.

▶ NURSING DIAGNOSIS: *Impaired Social Interaction*

Related To
- Maladaptive reaction to an identifiable stressor
- Situational and/or developmental crises
- Inadequate support systems

Defining Characteristics
- Feelings of isolation
- Depressed mood
- Lack of social outlets and support system

Patient Outcomes
Patient will demonstrate positive socialization patterns by the end of treatment.

Nursing Interventions	Rationales
Assess patient's available support system; focus interventions around making the support system more accessible so that it will better meet the patient's needs.	A positive and available support system can greatly assist the individual in coping with stress and stressful life events. Often in crisis periods, the support system cannot be accessed or is unavailable to the patient, thus making the crisis worse. The nurse can explore the support system with the patient and intervene where appropriate; for example, the nurse can suggest ways to broaden the support system or help the patient to make better use out of existing ones through a series of family/significant other meetings between the nurse, patient, and family/significant others.
Assist patient in developing social outlets and support systems to provide ego-enhancing experiences and relaxation.	Often when a maladaptive reaction to a psychosocial stressor is experienced, the patient becomes depressed and socially isolated, compounding the feelings of depression. It is important to encourage the patient to develop social outlets to mitigate against these feelings of social isolation and to encourage the development of adequate support systems.

CONTINUITY OF CARE/DISCHARGE PLANNING

- Refer for outpatient psychiatric care in the community in the form of individual, group, and/or family psychotherapy (depending upon the patient's unique circumstances).
- Encourage involvement in supportive relationships in the community (i.e., support groups, church activities, family functions, community involvement, volunteer activities, neighbors, friends, activities through community organizations such as the local mental health center, etc.).

BIBLIOGRAPHY

American Psychiatric Association (APA). (1994). *Diagnostic and statistical manual of mental disorders* (4th ed.). Washington, DC: APA.

Baier, M. (1987/1988). The "holiday blues" as a stress reaction. *Perspectives in Psychiatric Care, 24*(2), 64–68.

Gordon, M. (1991). *Manual of nursing diagnostics 1991–1992.* St. Louis, MO: Mosby-Year Book.

Kaplan, H., & Sadock, B. (1988). *Synopsis of psychiatry: Behavioral sciences, clinical psychiatry.* Baltimore, MD: Williams & Wilkins.

North American Nursing Diagnosis Association (NANDA). (1990). *NANDA nursing diagnosis: Definitions and classifications.* St. Louis, MO: NANDA.

Pickwell, S. (1989). The incorporation of family primary care for southeast Asian refugees in a community-based mental health facility. *Archives of Psychiatric Nursing, 3*(3), 173–177.

Townsend, M. C. (1988). *Nursing diagnosis in psychiatric nursing.* Philadelphia, PA: Davis.

Personality Disorders

Marga Simon Coler, EdD, RN, CS, CTN, FAAN

Personality Disorders are deviations of behaviors and inner experiences from one's cultural expectations. These personality traits are inflexible and maladaptive. The disorders must be visible in adolescence or early adulthood, become stable, and ultimately cause personal distress and impaired occupational and/or social functioning. Personality disorders persist throughout the adult life. They are generally ego dyntonic, which leads the person to seek therapeutic intervention. When they are ego syntonic, intervention becomes very difficult. Whether the disorder is ego systonic or ego dystonic, the individual is often aware of and dissatisfied with the impact that his or her inability to function effectively is having on others. Personality Disorders are grouped into three clusters: Cluster A individuals (Paranoid, Schizoid, and Schizotypal Personality Disorders) are eccentric or odd. Cluster B individuals (Antisocial, Borderline, Histrionic, and Narcissistic Disorders) appear erratic, dramatic, or emotional. Cluster C individuals (Avoidant, Passive-Aggressive, Dependent, or Obsessive-Compulsive Personality Disorders) are fearful and anxious. Personality Disorders not Otherwise Specified apply to individuals who do not meet the above-cited criteria.

The nursing syndrome characterizing Personality Disorders may therefore be defined as a malfunction in an individual's ability to relate to others based on non-reality-based thinking and distorted perceptions, which in turn cause an identity confusion. Ethnicity, culture, and social background must be considered in diagnostic formulation. The nursing syndrome evolves from the human response patterns (HRPs) relating, perceiving, valuing, and knowing and may be depicted as follows:

HRP	Nursing Diagnosis	Related To
Relating	Impaired social interaction	Sociocultural dissonance (i.e., behaviors or traits not accepted within sociocultural norms)
Perceiving	Personal identity disturbance	Inability to distinguish between the drives and boundaries of ego, libido, and superego
Valuing	Spiritual distress	Dissonance between societal/cultural value/belief system and that of self because of fluid ego boundaries
Knowing	Altered thought processes	Cognitive dissonance between sociocultural norms and those of the self

Nursing Interventions	Rationales
Assess for perceptual malfunctions.	Perceptual incoherence may contribute to misperceptions.
Establish a trusting relationship.	Individuals with personality disorders always have relationship problems.
Initiate individual psychotherapy.	Individuals with personality disorders do not function well in a group.
Teach strategies of conflict resolution.	The individual with a personality disorder has an inherent inability to delimit perceptions.
Teach strategies of values clarification.	An ability to sort values may help to achieve a normal balance between life experiences and instinctual needs.

Nursing Interventions	Rationales
Teach additional coping skills.	Certain coping defenses are used to excess, exaggerating or diminishing functioning.
Teach strategies of communication.	Socially appropriate communication is a learned behavior.

$\mathcal{P}$ARANOID PERSONALITY DISORDER

Marga Simon Coler, EdD, RN, CS, CTN, FAAN

Beginning at early adulthood, there is a persistent, ungrounded tendency to view the actions of others as threatening and belittling. The individual consistently senses exploitation by others. This is linked with pathological jealousy. These individuals are frequently aware that their ideas are considered unusual by associates; therefore, the personality may be hard to detect. Frequently the individual manages to go through life undiagnosed. However, at times, the symptoms become exaggerated to the extent that they may bring on other emotional disorders.

Clinical Clip

Many clinical characteristics of the individual with a Paranoid Personality Disorder are an exaggeration of the ego defense, projection.

ETIOLOGIES
(There is no information available).

CLINICAL MANIFESTATIONS
- Suspicious
- Perceives unapparent attacks by others
- Unforgiving
- Preoccupation with mistrust of others
- Reads threatening and demeaning hidden meanings into benign communication
- Doubts trustworthiness and sincerity of others
- Bears grudges
- Defensiveness

- Anger
- Hypervigilance
- Hostility
- Stubbornness
- Argumentative
- Exaggeration of incidents
- Reading of hidden meanings into the acts of others

- Sense of pride in being objective, rational, and without emotional involvement counterbalanced by a fear of loss of independence and powerlessness
- Relationships with others impaired

CLINICAL/DIAGNOSTIC FINDINGS
- Ideas of reference
- Antisocial traits

▶ NURSING DIAGNOSIS: *Impaired Social Interaction*
Related To a continuous sense of suspiciousness and distrust.

Defining Characteristics
- Suspiciousness
- Distrust
- Bears grudges
- Anger
- Hostile

- Unforgiving
- Easily offended
- Eccentric
- Serious, no sense of humor

Patient Outcomes
Patient will
- have a measure of insight into his or her condition.
- control impulses.
- seek socializing activities.
- have a sense of control over life.

Nursing Interventions	Rationales
Encourage socialization in task groups.	In task groups the ego boundaries are not threatened.
Encourage involvement in object-centered activities.	Since human relations are difficult to maintain, involvement with people in activities dealing with objects will provide socialization with minimal interaction.

▶ NURSING DIAGNOSIS: *Spiritual Distress*

Related To an inherent knowledge that they cannot relate to anyone, including significant others, without being suspicious of their actions.

Defining Characteristics
• Verbalizes inner conflicts about thoughts regarding motives of others
• Questions the loyalty of family, friends, and associates
• Questions the fidelity of sexual partner
• Is unforgiving
• Displaces anger toward clergy and other religious workers
• Is reluctant to confide in others

Patient Outcomes
Patient will
• gain a measure of insight into the etiology of the distress.
• gain a measure of tranquillity.
• achieve a personal sense of purpose to life.

Nursing Interventions	Rationales
Assess for cues relating to the spiritual aspects of patient's life.	Assessment provides cues on which to base therapy.
Initiate one-to-one therapy to explore the spiritual aspects of patient's life.	Awareness can, in itself, be curative.
Initiate values clarification therapy.	Since paranoid thinking and the resultant spiritual distress are generally not amenable to therapy, a sorting of values may provide a recipe for dealing with the mental anguish.
Initiate behavior modification as needed.	Since it is difficult to affect the distress of paranoid thinking through insight, the modification of behavior toward cultural acceptance may be an alternative toward its alleviation.

▶ NURSING DIAGNOSIS: *Powerlessness*

Related To a perceived lack of control over environment.

Defining Characteristics
- Expressions of lack of control
- Passivity
- Reluctance (inability?) to express feelings
- Anger
- Misconstrued apprehensions

Patient Outcomes
Patient will
- exercise control over thought processes.
- modify verbal communication so as not to offend others.
- learn to establish a trusting relationship with at least one significant other.

Nursing Interventions	Rationales
Provide opportunities for freedom of choice.	There is a prevailing suspicion that others are trying to control.
Do not argue with patient.	Arguing threatens autonomy.
Encourage expressing perceptions of powerlessness to therapist when they arise.	A psychotherapist can help patient conquer the feeling of powerlessness.

▶ NURSING DIAGNOSIS: *Personal Identity Disturbance*

Related To an inability to actualize the self instead of a self-image based on perceptions of what others think.

Defining Characteristics
- Apparent reality confusion
- Feeling of isolation
- Apparent identity confusion
- Apparent loss of ego boundaries
- Reading threatening and/or demeaning meanings into everyday remarks by others
- Expecting exploitation or harm from others
- Misinterpretation of thoughts of others
- Interjection of environmental input rather than assimilation
- Projection of thoughts

Patient Outcomes
Patient will have an awareness of
- his or her identity.
- biopsychospiritual boundaries.
- the mechanisms of introjection and projection.

Nursing Interventions	Rationales
Initiate one-to-one psycho-therapeutic intervention using techniques of 1. reality-orientation. 2. nondirective intervention. 3. behavior modification. 4. values clarification. 5. cognitive therapy.	One-to-one therapy will help build trust and confidence where there is a loss of ego boundaries; group or family therapy could be overwhelming. 1. This will help to sort out facts from erroneous beliefs about situations. 2. The patient continues to assume charge of his or her life with guidance from nurse. Roles are clarified in this manner. 3. The patient is taught to change from nonadaptive to adaptive behavior in spite of paranoid thought process. This in turn will strengthen self-identity. 4. The clarification of a value system will serve to strengthen ego boundaries. 5. Learning about the mechanisms of introjection and projection may lead to adaptive behavior, which in turn will serve to strengthen ego boundaries by providing guidelines for ego performance.

▶ NURSING DIAGNOSIS: *Ineffective Individual Coping*

Related To unusual ideas and extreme behaviors.

Defining Characteristics
- Impaired social participation
- Self-destructive behavior
- Self-destructive thought patterns
- Inherent misinterpretation of actions and thoughts of others as demeaning and/or threatening
- Projection
- Disturbances of mood

Patient Outcomes
Patient will
- define adaptive responses.
- modify maladaptive responses.

Nursing Interventions	Rationales
Assess for maladaptive responses.	Identification of maladaptive responses will help the process of acknowledgment which must occur before replacement can occur.
Initiate one-to-one psychotherapeutic intervention using: 1. nondirective intervention. 2. behavior modification. 3. values clarification. 4. cognitive therapy.	One-to-one intervention will aid in building trust and confidence, which will enhance the exchanging of maladaptive for adaptive coping skills. 1. The patient continues to assume charge of his or her life with guidance from nurse. The active identification of maladaptive coping strategies by the patient will ultimately enhance their replacement by adaptive coping strategies. 2. Since there is very little insight because of paranoid thought processes, the patient can learn to replace maladaptive coping strategies by adaptive ones. 3. The clarification of values will serve to strengthen ego boundaries. 4. Learning about the mechanisms of ego defense will aid in the replacement of maladaptive by adaptive behavior, which in turn will serve to strengthen ego boundaries by providing guidelines for ego performance.

CONTINUITY OF CARE/DISCHARGE PLANNING
- Maintain monthly visits as needed to help patient base distorted perceptions on reality.

BIBLIOGRAPHY
American Psychiatric Association (APA). (1994). *Diagnostic and statistical manual of mental disorders* (4th ed.). Washington, DC: APA.

Burgess, A. (1990). *Psychiatric nursing in the hospital and the community.* Norwalk, CT: Appleton & Lange.

Danaher-Dunn, P. (1992). Social interaction, impaired. In K. Gettrust & P. Brabec (Eds.), *Nursing diagnosis in clinical practice.* Albany, NY: Delmar.

Fitzpatrick, J. (1991). Taxonomy II: Definitions and development. In R. Carroll-Johnson (Ed.), *Classification of nursing diagnoses. Proceedings of the Ninth Conference of the North American Nursing Diagnosis Association.* Philadelphia, PA: Lippincott.

Houseman, C. (1990). The paranoid person: A biopsychosocial perspective. *Archives of Psychiatric Nursing, IV,* 176–182.

Koneazny, K. (1992). Coping, impaired individual. In K. Gettrust & P. Brabec (Eds.), *Nursing diagnosis in clinical practice.* Albany, NY: Delmar.

North American Nursing Diagnosis Association (NANDA). (1992). *NANDA nursing diagnoses: Definitions and classification 1992.* St. Louis, MO: NANDA.

Slimmer, L. (1992). Powerlessness. In K. Gettrust & P. Brabec (Eds.), *Nursing diagnosis in clinical practice.* Albany, NY: Delmar.

Task Force on *DSM-IV,* American Psychiatric Association (APA). (1993). *DSM-IV draft criteria.* Washington, DC: APA.

Valentin, C. (1992). Personal identity disturbance. In K. Gettrust & P. Brabec (Eds.), *Nursing diagnosis in clinical practice.* Albany, NY: Delmar.

VandeVusse, L. (1992). Spiritual distress. In K. Gettrust & P. Brabec (Eds.), *Nursing diagnosis in clinical practice.* Albany, NY: Delmar.

ANTISOCIAL PERSONALITY DISORDERS

Eileen Tarsky, BSN, RN, C

The Antisocial Personality Disorder is defined as a consistent pattern of irresponsible and antisocial behavior since the age of 15. The individual must be at least 18 years of age at the time this diagnosis is made. These individuals have limited experience and expression of emotions. This disorder is more frequent in males and very difficult to treat. Society has usually used incarceration as a mode of containment.

ETIOLOGIES
- Possible involvement of genetic factors [some studies have shown that parents of individuals with this disorder have exhibited excessive electroencephalogram (EEG) abnormalities]
- Parental abandonment and abuse
- Inconsistent or harsh punishment by parents
- Absence of discipline
- Never having to suffer the consequence of their own behavior (being rescued)
- Parental rejection
- Brain injury or head trauma may predispose

CLINICAL MANIFESTATIONS
- Inability to sustain satisfactory job performance
- Inability to develop satisfying, enduring, intimate relationships with others
- Failure to follow social and legal norms; repeated performance of antisocial acts which are grounds for arrest
- Repeated failure to meet financial obligations
- Impulsivity (extreme)/poor frustration tolerance
- Lack of guilt and remorse
- Repeated lying and conning of others for self-satisfying gains

- Aggressiveness, may be physically violent
- Generalized irritability
- Abuse of others to validate own superiority
- Evidence of Conduct Disorder with onset before age 15 years

CLINICAL/DIAGNOSTIC FINDINGS
Patient should have a thorough physical examination and history to rule out a physiological cause for violence such as frontal lobe injury or other brain lesions:
- physical
  - low level of autonomic arousal
  - abnormal EEG—higher amounts of slow wave activity which may reflect a deficit in inhibitory mechanisms
  - average to above average intelligence on psychological testing
- psychological
  - displays lack of emotional attachment
  - preoccupation with self and needs
  - grandiose sense of own importance
  - low frustration tolerance
  - projects responsibility of life circumstance upon others
  - need for immediate gratification
  - erratic and extreme expression of emotions

▶ NURSING DIAGNOSIS: *High Risk for Violence—Directed at Others*

Risk Factors
- Antisocial character
- Rage (easily accessible)
- Diminished frustration tolerance
- Substance abuse
- Learned behavior
- Past utilization of assaults when angry
- Body language which exhibits muscle tension/intense effort to control (e.g., clenching hands, jaw tightening)
- Boasting of past abuse to others
- Possession of destructive means: gun, knife, other weapon
- Hostility, may be provocative during verbal interaction, threatening

Patient Outcomes
Patient will
- identify situations which may precipitate hostility (rage, acting out).
- acknowledge responsibility to maintain control over behavior.
- learn to verbalize needs with nonaggressive behaviors.
Patient, others, and staff will remain free from harm.

Nursing Interventions	Rationales
Provide and convey a trusting and consistent attitude by speaking in a calm manner. Resist responding to provocative behavior or verbalizations of anger.	Promotes self-worth and provides basis for therapeutic relationship. May change the style of relating and provide opportunity for constructive change in relationships.
Assess and document past history of violent behavior.	Team needs to be aware of style of acting-out behavior(s) to provide safety for individual and others (e.g., events that precipitate violent outbursts).
Observe patient's behavior frequently. Be aware of escalating behaviors (e.g., clenched fist, tautness).	Team can intervene before situation escalates to one of violence.
Remove all dangerous objects from environment.	Objects cannot be used as weapons against self or others.
Assist in identifying the true object of their hostility.	Displacement of anger can be an inappropriate use of defense mechanisms.
Encourage verbalization of feelings.	Verbalization increases self-awareness between feelings and behaviors.
Help to find alternative methods of expression for anger and hostility (e.g., physical exercise, relaxation, and assertiveness training).	Alternate coping skills are essential to break the maladaptive pattern of responding to stress and unmet needs.

▶ NURSING DIAGNOSIS: *Self-Esteem Disturbance*

Related To
- Unmet dependency needs
- Dysfunctional family system
- Retarded ego development
- Lack of positive feedback

Defining Characteristics
- Projection of blame/responsibility for problems
- Aggressive behavior
- Critical of others and use of derogatory comments against them
- Use of manipulation
- Acting-out behaviors [e.g., ethyl alcohol (ETOH)/substance abuse, sexual promiscuity]

Patient Outcomes

Patient will

- recognize need for change in behaviors and verbalize responsibility taking for this action.
- recognize that the use of derogatory comments toward others is a reflection of his or her own poor self-esteem.
- verbalize enhanced self-esteem by conversing without using self-negating comments.

Nursing Interventions	Rationales
Assist in setting reasonable and obtainable goals.	Success in achieving treatment goals is enabled and a positive self-regard enhanced.
Assist in identifying positive aspects of self.	Self-reflection and mastery over self-esteem are encouraged.
Identify manipulative behavior and establish behavioral contract.	This assists in reality testing when behaviors or verbal dialogue is counterproductive.
Minimize negative feedback and enforce limit setting in matter-of-fact way.	The therapeutic interaction objective is maintained and focused on positive observations of behavior.
Assist patient to enhance social participation via development of new interpersonal skills; use positive feedback for appropriate interactions.	When dealing with a set of unproductive and even self-destructive behaviors, social and coping skills training is often necessary.
Teach assertiveness skills/techniques, especially the difference between assertiveness and aggressiveness. Identify the need to demonstrate respect for all individuals, including self.	Use of cognitive techniques assists in improving self-esteem and relationship to others.

▶ NURSING DIAGNOSIS: *Ineffective Individual Coping*

Related To

- Lack of role models
- Inadequate support systems
- Inadequate methods of coping
- Inability to experience guilt/shame as an internal monitor for behaviors

Defining Characteristics
- Substance abuse
- Impulsive acts of violence
- Socially unacceptable behavior on a continued basis
- Inability to maintain employment and relationships

Patient Outcomes
Patient will
- identify past methods and outcome of coping.
- verbalize the need to explore and adapt new methods of coping.
- demonstrate these new methods in therapeutic milieu activities and groups.

Nursing Interventions	Rationales
Establish regular meeting time on a daily basis.	Boundaries are set around the therapeutic relationship and consistency in schedule is taught.
Review past antisocial/acting-out behavior and impact on life/relationships.	A baseline assessment of deficits is established in coping/relating skills and a mirror to view cause and effect of behavior provided.
Explore alternative methods of coping which might have been used and the possible outcome(s).	This assists in identifying new ways of dealing with stress and/or relationships.
Encourage to keep a notebook of feelings and angry/hostile thoughts and the situation which provoked them. Review regularly and have the patient suggest alternative reactions/responses.	This exercise will glean information about triggers for aggressive/hostile thoughts and actions, the underlying feelings, and reactions. It can provide a sense of control over finding alternatives to usual methods of dealing with situations.
Provide groups as a forum for emotional expression and reality testing.	A group provides an avenue for practicing new coping and interpersonal skills in a safe and structured setting.
Encourage attendance at Alcoholics Anonymous and/or Narcotics Anonymous meetings.	Peer support and pressure are highly successful in dealing with acting-out behavior.
Recognize appropriate coping skills with positive feedback.	The internalization of coping skills and a positive self-regard are reinforced.

▶ NURSING DIAGNOSIS: *Dysfunctional Grieving*

Related To
- Deprivation of basic needs (e.g., shelter, food, clothing, love, safety)
- Unavailable support system
- Lack of consistent parental involvement
- Lack of emotional availability of caretakers

Defining Characteristics
- Denial of loss
- Developmental regression
- Interference with life functions
- Difficulty expressing the meaning of loss

Patient Outcomes
Patient will
- identify true source of anger.
- actualize loss and progress through the grieving process (this is a long process and patient will require long-term outpatient therapy).

Nursing Interventions	Rationales
Assist to identify the multiple losses/deprivations in life.	The process of review of the life story and identification of multiple losses is begun.
Establish an accepting, nonthreatening relationship by being honest and caring.	A nonthreatening interaction sets a model for a new type of trusting relationship, thus encouraging honest and vulnerable sharing.
Assist in identifying the emotional impact of the loss.	Patient can begin to work through the grieving process.
Explore feelings and true source of anger (e.g., maternal deprivation).	This role models appropriate avenues for expression of anger and acceptance of negative feelings, which can allow internal forgiveness.
Set clear expectations of behavioral controls and provide limit setting.	The expectation that grief can be tolerated within the therapy is defined and responsibility of control is placed with the client.

CONTINUITY OF CARE/DISCHARGE PLANNING

- Refer to residential program, Alcoholics Anonymous, Narcotics Anonymous, and outpatient therapy.

BIBLIOGRAPHY

Burgess, A. W. (1990). *Psychiatric nursing in the hospital and the community.* Norwalk, CT: Appleton & Lange.

Gordon, M. (1993). *Manual of nursing diagnosis.* New York: McGraw-Hill.

Haber, J., Hoskins, P., Leach, A., & Sideleau, B. (1987). *Comprehensive psychiatric nursing.* New York: McGraw-Hill.

Task Force on *DSM-IV*, American Psychiatric Association (APA). (1991). *DSM-IV options book: Work in progress.* Washington, DC: APA.

Townsend, M. (1991). *Nursing diagnosis in psychiatric nursing.* Philadelphia: Davis.

$\mathcal{B}$ORDERLINE PERSONALITY DISORDER

Christine Fitzpatrick, MS, RN, CS

The diagnosis Borderline Personality Disorder (BPD) is one that stirs up great controversy among both theorists and clinicians. It is a term that is often overused and frequently carries a pejorative connotation. Patients diagnosed with BPD are challenging to treat in light of their unique configuration of dysfunctional reality interpretations and coping strategies, possibly including transference of feelings of rage or rescue onto the caregiver. A difficult patient can easily be diagnosed with BPD, when, in fact, he or she may suffer from an underlying affective disorder. On the other hand, an individual with BPD can present with a very complex constellation of symptoms, including social skills, which are used to keep people away, thus making it difficult to diagnose BPD.

Clinical Clip

After a thorough assessment of the patient, the clinician is usually left with a number of competing differential diagnoses, including Major Depression with Psychotic or Suicidal features, Schizotypal Personality, a Primary Addictive or Eating Disorder, and Adjustment Reaction or Posttraumatic Stress Syndrome.

ETIOLOGIES
- Failure in successful completion of the reproachment, or separation, phase during childhood, leaving the child with a poor sense of self and highly vulnerable to separation anxiety or panic
- Genetic theory: vulnerability to stressful situations, intolerance to physical and emotional symptoms of anxiety and poor impulse control, leading to a tendency toward extreme rage reactions

- Experienced family violence, drug or alcohol abuse of one or both parents, and physical, sexual, and/or emotional abuse

CLINICAL MANIFESTATIONS
- Unstable and intense interpersonal relationships marked by extremes of overidealization or devaluation of the person
- Impulsive in at least two areas that are potentially self-damaging, e.g., spending, sex, substance use, shoplifting, reckless driving, and binge eating
- Lability of mood; shifts between depression, irritability, or anxiety, usually lasting a few hours
- Inappropriate, intense anger or lack of control of anger
- Recurrent suicidal threats, gestures, or behavior or self-mutilating behavior
- Marked and persistent identity disturbance manifested by uncertainty about sexual orientation, long-term goals or career choice, type of friends desired, and preferred values
- Chronic feelings of emptiness or boredom
- Frantic efforts to avoid real or imagined abandonment
- Inability to tolerate ambivalent feelings toward people

CLINICAL/DIAGNOSTIC FINDINGS
- Intense affect, usually of a strongly hostile or depressed nature. The absence of pleasure and the presence of depersonalization may be useful in differential diagnosis.
- A history of impulsive behavior, including both episodic acts (e.g., self-mutilation, overdose of drugs) and more chronic behavior patterns (e.g., drug dependence, promiscuity). Often the result of these behaviors is self-destructive although their purpose is not.
- Apparent social adaptiveness (good achievement in school or work, appropriate appearance and manners, and strong social awareness), which masks mimicry (rapid and superficial identification with others).
- Brief psychotic experiences, specifically, paranoid features.
- Psychological testing performance: evidence of bizarre, dereistic, illogical, or primitive responses on unstructured tests such as the Rorschach; positive neurotic and psychotic evaluation on the Minnesota Multiphasic Personality Inventory Scale
- Interpersonal relationships, which vacillate between transient and superficial relationships and intense, dependent relationships that are marred by devaluation, manipulation, and demandingness
- Hypochondriosis or somatization of symptoms
- Eating disorders
- Intolerance of being alone
- Low achievement despite intellectual capabilities
- Physician shopping

▶ NURSING DIAGNOSIS: *Anxiety*

Related To

- Unconscious conflict about values/goals of life
- Perceived threats to self-concept
- Anticipated threats of abandonment by significant others
- Unmet needs
- Inability to voice feelings

Defining Characteristics

- Increased tension
- Painful and persistent increased helplessness
- Verbalizations of being scared
- Shakiness
- Regretful
- Distressed
- Apprehensive/fearful
- Feelings of uncertainty/inadequacy
- Fear of unspecified consequences
- Somatic complaints
- Sense of impending doom
- Somatic symptoms, i.e., rapid pulse, rapid heart rate, shortness of breath, poor eye contact, quivering voice, potential self-mutilation

Patient Outcomes

Patient will

- learn strategies of relaxation.
- learn to identify and express different emotions.
- express decreased symptoms of anxiety.

Nursing Interventions	Rationales
Conduct a thorough nursing history, including a physical exam.	A history rules out physiological causes for symptoms and provides insight into interpersonal and social causes of anxiety symptoms
Determine subjective experience of anxiety; both somatic and emotional feelings.	This helps to determine contact with and ability to verbally express emotions that may present as anxiety.
Review present methods of dealing with anxiety, especially use of self-mutilation.	Identifying the present methods of dealing with anxiety, especially harmful ones, allows teaching about stress and coping and thus avoiding feelings of shame/guilt.
Speak in a calm manner, using short, simple sentences.	Calmness is conveyed in a verbal manner. Also, high-anxiety states interfere with cognitive functioning, and speaking with short,

Nursing Interventions	Rationales
	simple words will convey the message more directly.
Review with the patient a mutually agreed-upon plan of care.	Patient involvement in and agreement with goals and approach foster sense of control and increase compliance.
Choose an initial selection of concrete goals.	This will help focus the therapy and minimize the difficulty the borderline patient has with intimacy and trust
Teach relaxation techniques such as guided imagery, meditation, deep breathing, or progressive relaxation.	Active relaxation techniques will help with anxiety reduction and control.
Set clear limits about availability outside of therapeutic sessions and time limits surrounding the therapy sessions at the start.	Limits may be tested in an effort to determine the therapist's reliability and caring.
The therapist must monitor his or her own affect and emotional experience.	A therapist's strong reaction to some aspect of the patient's behavior can provide valuable information about the patient if it can be understood.
The therapist should resist responding to each new symptom as an emergency.	Many of the problems will be transitory; focusing on each event diverts from the course of treatment.
Evaluate the effectiveness of the interventions via reports of anxiety reactions.	Active relaxation interventions and movement toward understanding causes of anxiety (underlying unresolved or unacknowledged feelings) will decrease anxiety levels.

▶ NURSING DIAGNOSIS: *Ineffective Individual Coping*

Related To
- Personal vulnerability
- Inadequate role models

- Dysfunctional family system
- Lack of pertinent knowledge

Defining Characteristics
- Inability to meet role expectations

- Inability to problem solve

- Alteration in societal participation
- Inappropriate use of defense mechanisms
- Verbal manipulation
- High illness rate
- High rate of accidents

- Overeating
- Excessive drinking and/or smoking
- Overuse of prescribed tranquilizers
- Destructive behavior toward self or others

Patient Outcomes

Patient will

- learn strategies for reality testing, especially in interpersonal relationships.
- learn to tolerate intense emotions.
- begin to accept and acknowledge responsibility for own behavior.
- exhibit alternative ways of dealing with negative feelings.
- attend to instructions given by one staff person at a time.
- communicate needs, frustrations, and feelings in constructive verbal ways to staff.

Nursing Interventions	Rationales
Assess present coping methods used during therapy and in unit milieu.	A baseline of coping mechanisms is established, which can be used to measure growth and expansion of styles of coping.
Identify present stressors.	Severity and/or number of stressors in life can compromise coping techniques. Interventions may have to be tailored to help adjust to current stressful events.
Focus attention on behaviors and reactions to stress events, rather than helping place blame for the incident. Relay perceptions in a clear, descriptive, and nonjudgmental manner.	Patient is encouraged to own behaviors and response to stressors and to view coping styles without shame or guilt.
Assess response to limits within the therapy and on the unit.	Effectiveness of limit setting is determined.
After superficial goals are met, begin in-depth work regarding dichotomous thinking.	Small successes will build trust in the therapeutic relationship and prepare for more difficult task of looking critically at dysfunctional thinking patterns and resultant behavior.

Nursing Interventions	Rationales
Work at critically looking at difficult situations as they arise and help develop useful problem-solving techniques.	This activity will help reduce the intensity of emotional responses to events after the fact.
Assist to identify subjective experience of emotional turmoil.	Usual manner of response to emotional turmoil is impulsive activity. If patients can learn to recognize internal turmoil, they can interrupt impulsive reactions and replace them with constructive methods of dealing with the problem.
Encourage role playing/rehearsing of constructive coping mechanisms.	Patient can learn new methods of dealing with stress.
Provide positive feedback for new coping skills training.	Positive changes are encouraged and feelings of self-mastery enhanced.
Encourage interaction in groups on the unit to facilitate social situations, where new coping techniques may be practiced.	The repertoire of coping skills is enlarged to include social interaction skills.
Evaluate utilization and success of new coping strategies.	Evaluation of intervention and feedback to patient will build feelings of success and provide insight into changing other coping mechanisms.

▶ NURSING DIAGNOSIS: *Posttrauma Response*

Related To past history of physical, emotional, and/or sexual abuse.

Defining Characteristics
- Psychic/emotional numbness
  - impaired interpretation of reality
  - dissociation
- Self-destructiveness
- Detachment
- Poor impulse control
- Irritability and explosiveness
- Social dependence, isolation, or avoidance

Patient Outcomes
Patient will
- integrate the traumatic event into life story without further symptoms.

- begin to develop support system of trusting relationships with men and women.

Nursing Interventions	Rationales
Assess the nature of the past abuse.	A history of past abuse determines whether the abuse was physical, emotional, and/or sexual in nature and ascertains the emotional impact of abuse.
Determine the response to the event both currently and in the past.	The emotional impact of the abuse on current functioning is reviewed.
Assess whether there is any current contact with the perpetrator and the nature of the relationship.	If there is current contact with the perpetrator, the nature of the relationship may be exacerbating the symptoms and delaying the healing process.
Ascertain the coping mechanisms used to deal with the memories of the trauma.	This determines whether positive or negative coping mechanisms are being used, such as drinking, self-mutilation, eating disorders, and provides directions for further clinical interventions.
Remind that flashbacks may be memories of emotions as well as of physical acts.	During the life review part of therapy patient is reassured that the flashbacks are memories of the past and not reoccurring in the present. A sense of safety is maintained.
Provide the opportunity to relate the story of the abuse, including the emotions involved. Assure that the therapy happens in a safe, structured setting and that the patient has social/emotional support after the session.	The individual is allowed to relate details of the event and the emotions involved in a supportive environment. This experience may be the first time that he or she has had the opportunity to tell someone who would believe the story. If inpatient, provide emotional support (sometimes just a reassuring physical presence) after the session, if required.
Allow the unfoldment of memories and emotions at the individual's own pace. Reassure patient that therapy will only proceed at that pace.	Patient is reassured that he or she will not be overwhelmed by emotions.

Nursing Interventions	Rationales
Continually check for safety issues.	Whether the patient is becoming overwhelmed is evaluated.
Reorient to place, person, and time at end of session.	Disorientation may occur when relating intensely emotionally charged events from the past.
Provide emotional support on the unit if life review work is being done in individual or group therapy.	Continued safety during hospitalization and between sessions is ensured.
Evaluate extent of intrusion of thoughts about event into daily life.	The effectiveness of the intervention is evaluated.

▶ NURSING DIAGNOSIS: *High Risk for Self-Mutilation*

Risk Factors
- Diagnosis of BPD
- History of self-injury
- History of physical, emotional, and/or sexual abuse
- Inability to cope with increased psychological/physiological tension in a healthy manner
- Feelings of depression, rejection, self-hatred, separation anxiety, guilt, and depersonalization
- Dysfunctional family of origin

Patient Outcomes
Patient will
- exhibit constructive methods of dealing with perceived rejection, stress, or anxiety without hurting self.
- contract for safety with health care providers.

Nursing Interventions	Rationales
Assess past experiences with self-mutilating behavior, i.e., timing, preceding events, severity of injury, and ability to contact health care providers.	A history establishes baseline data of lethality of past episodes of self-mutilation, events preceding the act, and ability to establish trusting relationship with health care providers.

Nursing Interventions	Rationales
Ascertain patient's insights into causes and consequences of self-destructive behavior.	Patient's ability to identify emotional situations that can escalate negative self-destructive behavior is determined.
Evaluate social support system available.	Positive social support can be a critical element in the holistic care plan for a patient; it provides reality testing, safety, and positive regard.
Design a plan of contracting for safety or contacting health care providers (both inpatient and outpatient) if feelings of self-mutilation increase.	Health care providers and patient act as a team in identifying predictors for increased risk for self-harm and plans to follow to access the health care system.
Monitor ability to follow through with plan during course of treatment.	This provides ongoing assessment of ability to contract and incidence of self-mutilating vs. constructive means of dealing with negative emotions.

▶ NURSING DIAGNOSIS: *Impaired Social Interaction*

Related To
- Knowledge/skill deficit about ways to relate
- Self-concept disturbance
- Absence of role models
- Past history of abusive relationships

Defining Characteristics
- Verbalized or observed discomfort in social situations
- Verbalized or observed inability to receive or communicate a satisfying sense of belonging, caring, interest, or shared history
- Observed use of unsuccessful social interaction skills
- Dysfunctional interaction with peers, family, and/or others

Patient Outcomes
Patient will
- demonstrate new positive relationships.
- express difficulties encountered in social relationships rather than abandoning the relationship.
- begin to identify and accept pros and cons of relationships.

Nursing Interventions	Rationales
Assess and document past experiences of social activities and interaction.	This helps to identify previous level of functioning and types of activities enjoyed.
Assess current strengths and problem areas regarding social interactions.	This identifies areas of strength to reinforce and build upon, as well as problem areas that can be improved.
Identify, with the patient, goals for increased social interaction.	Mutually agreed-upon goals will be more easily attained.
Support and reinforce efforts and successes in social interactions (be specific regarding the situations to be reinforced).	Positive reinforcement, even for approximations of what is expected, can be very reinforcing and encouraging for patients who are trying to master change in behavior.
Teach components of appropriate social interaction. Social skills include eye contact, speech, and how (behaviorally) to relate a message.	Normalizes social skills deficit as a learned behavior and engages patient in treatment process.
Provide emotional support as skills are practiced toward achievement of goals.	Low self-esteem may result in discouragement about performance of new skills or reactions of others to efforts to socialize and communicate. Empathetic listening and support can help them to continue their efforts.
Provide a group situation to improve social skills.	An opportunity to practice skills in a nonthreatening situation is provided.
Evaluate the care as needed to ensure the direction and method of treatment are appropriate.	Evaluation of care needed ensures that goals are neither too advanced nor too slow for patient's needs and that opportunities for skill development match the needs.

▶ NURSING DIAGNOSIS: *Chronic Low Self-Esteem*

Related To:
- History of physical or emotional abuse
- Inadequate role models
- Dysfunctional family of origin

Defining Characteristics

- Verbalizes inability to deal with events
- Exaggerates negative feedback about the self
- Expresses shame or guilt
- Indecisive
- Minimizes or rationalizes away positive feedback
- Verbalizes self-negating or derogatory statements
- Hesitant to try new things or situations

Patient Outcomes

Patient will

- begin to make positive self-regard statements regarding strengths, capabilities, and talents.
- enter some new social/occupational situations without resulting injury to self.
- listen to positive feedback about job performance or activities in the milieu without self-negating remarks.

Nursing Interventions	Rationales
Assess for duration and perceived factors associated with low self-esteem.	Identification of duration and depth of problem and any associated problems is vital to planning care and promoting patient participation.
Initiate therapeutic relationship.	Acceptance and respect on the part of the nurse promote self-acceptance and growth.
Conduct a positive asset search.	Identifying assets serves to reinforce existing self-worth and identify strengths for treatment tasks.
Teach cognitive/behavioral skills of assertiveness and cognitive restructuring.	Increased assertion is likely to result in reinforcing feelings of competence. If negative self-talk reinforces low self-esteem or feelings of inadequacy, patients can be taught to replace these negative thoughts with realistic assessments of strengths.

CONTINUITY OF CARE/DISCHARGE PLANNING

- Arrange for weekly psychotherapy in either outpatient or inpatient settings. In more severe cases of BPD, the patient may require three to five visits a week.
- Advise that short hospitalizations may be required during highly stressful times in the patient's life. It is in their best interest to keep hospitalizations short as they can regress further in the hospital.

BIBLIOGRAPHY

American Psychiatric Association (APA). 1994. *Diagnostic and statistical manual of mental disorders* (4th ed.). Washington, DC: APA.

Beck, A., & Freeman A. (1992). *The cognitive therapy of borderline personality disorder.* New York: Guildford Publications.

Doenges, M., & Moorehouse, M. (1988). *Nursing diagnoses with interventions.* Philadelphia, PA: Davis.

Groves, J. (1981). Borderline personality disorder. *New England Journal of Medicine 305,* 259–262.

Gunderson, J., & Singer, M. (1975). *American Journal of Psychiatry, 132*(1), 1–20.

Kernberg, O. (1967). Borderline personality organization. *Journal of the American Psychoanalytic Association,* 150, 641–685.

Waldinger, R. J. (1986). Assessing borderline personality. *Medical Aspects of Human Sexuality, June,* 40–50.

OBSESSIVE-COMPULSIVE PERSONALITY DISORDER

Joan Bavoux, RN, C

Obsessive-Compulsive Personality Disorder (OCPD) is characterized by a life-long pattern or style of relating to the world in a rigid and inflexible manner. This behavioral style allows persons to perceive themselves as maintaining both mental and interpersonal control. The major behaviors utilized are a preoccupation with perfectionism, i.e., orderliness and cleanliness, and an obsession for detail in all their activities.

ETIOLOGIES
- Biological and developmental factors have not been specifically identified for the etiology of OCPD. However, several cognitive and psychoanalytic theories suggest causes for this personality development.
- Psychoanalytic theory suggests that strict, controlling, rigid, and punitive parenting during the bowel training period of psychosexual development results in extreme anxiety and frustration for the child. This trauma may result in the individual's overwhelming need to control his or her environment to the finest detail.
- Cognitive theory views OCPD as a set of misconceptions about expectations for behavior and life set by patients themselves.

CLINICAL MANIFESTATIONS
- Preoccupation with lists, rules, and details, resulting in loss of the major point of the activity
- Vivid imaginations
- Rigid perfectionism, e.g., often fail to complete projects because of inability to achieve high performance and outcome
- Heightened sense of responsibility

- Excessive preoccupation with work, when not economically necessary, to the detriment of social obligations
- Noncultural/religiously imposed inflexibility regarding ethics, morality, and values; overconscientiousness; scrupulousness
- Inability to accept change
- Poverty of warm emotions, hypersensitivity, lack of confidence, low self-esteem
- Inability to discard useless objects
- Reluctance to delegate related to feeling others cannot do assignment correctly or as well
- Hoarding of money for future catastrophe, miserly spending style toward self and others
- Inability to accept change
- Stubbornness, rigidity in interpersonal relationships
- Depressed mood with chronic worrying/extreme feelings of guilt
- Potential for major depression and/or anxiety disorders

CLINICAL/DIAGNOSTIC FINDINGS
(None)

▶ NURSING DIAGNOSIS: *Ineffective Individual Coping*

Related To personal vulnerability and rigid and inflexible orientation to life and others.

Defining Characteristics
- High illness or accident rate (insomnia, ulcers, hypertension, irritable bowel)
- Substance abuse
- Use of perfectionism; denial of fear, anxiety, and/or anger; projection; intellectualization
- Verbalization of inability to cope
- Inability to solve problems (procrastination, ambivalence)

Patient Outcomes
Patient will
- verbalize psychic discomfort and need for behavioral change.
- verbalize range of feelings.
- identify maladaptive coping patterns and consequences.
- identify strengths.
- identify goals and make decisions to actively pursue changes in life.
- identify needs for follow-up treatment.

Nursing Interventions	Rationales
Conduct a thorough physical and psychosocial history.	A baseline of coping mechanisms and behaviors that interfere with social and occupational life is established.
Assess for suicidality.	Increased awareness of impact of past behavior on quality of life may precipitate a major depression and suicidal ideation.
Assess sleep pattern, elimination, dietary intake, interests in pleasurable activities, and reasons for seeking treatment.	Data are useful to rule out or rule in vegetative signs of major depression.
Engage family/significant others in initial assessment.	Interactions with the family/significant others can give a valuable perspective on the quality of the relationship between the family and patient. Also, information about rituals and extent of striving for perfection vs. immobility of action are determined.
Encourage socialization through focused group activities, participation of family in passes, or therapy.	Activity can decrease anxiety and depressive symptoms, increase subjective feelings of connecting with others in a supportive environment, and continue or enhance the relationship within family.
Teach about substance use as an abuse of self.	Substance abuse is a short-term coping mechanism with long-term negative side effects. Education about alternative coping mechanisms to deal with feelings can empower the patient.
Teach problem-solving techniques.	Patient is encouraged to move through stages of problem identification, sorting through alternatives and choosing a solution, all goal-directed and action-oriented activities.
Teach stress reduction.	Positive techniques, such as yoga, meditation, breathing exercises,

Nursing Interventions	Rationales
	and exercise, decrease stress on a long-term basis.

▶ NURSING DIAGNOSIS: *Impaired Social Interaction*

Related To style of rigid perfectionism and need for detail, poor self-esteem, and poor social skills.

Defining Characteristics
- Social isolation
- Superficial relationships
- Verbalization of discomfort in social situations

Patient Outcomes
Patient will
- identify behaviors that interfere with social relationships.
- substitute constructive behaviors, i.e., complimenting others when appropriate.
- enlist significant others in promotion of effective socialization.

Nursing Interventions	Rationales
Explore quality of relationships at work, home, or school.	The environment where impaired social interactions occur is identified.
Assist in identifying present character of social relationships and goals for future relationships.	The problem-solving technique of specifically identifying the difficulties in a relationship and moving towards solutions is employed.
Provide assistance in decreasing life stresses which are present-oriented and based in reality. Help identify alternative coping mechanisms.	Appropriate social skills within the therapeutic alliance are taught; the emerging relationship can be used as an example of positive skill building.
Involve in a social skill-building environment group which includes education about social skills, role playing, peer support within the group, rehearsing behaviors, and	This provides a supportive environment to learn socialization skills needed for basic living, testing of new social skills, developing relationships within the

Nursing Interventions	Rationales
experiencing actual problem situations and solutions.	group, and ultimately, decreasing social isolation.
Evaluate new social skills.	Ongoing learning and practicing of positive social behaviors to decrease perception of isolation are encouraged.

► NURSING DIAGNOSIS: *Self-Esteem Disturbance*

Related To unrealistic expectations of self.

Defining Characteristics
- Hesitancy to try new things/situations
- Denial of problems apparent to others
- Projection of blame
- Rationalization of failure
- Hypersensitivity to slight or criticism
- Grandiosity
- Expression of shame/guilt

Patient Outcomes
Patient will
- identify positive and realistic perceptions of self.
- socialize with others in activities.
- begin to problem solve about dilemmas in life.

Nursing Interventions	Rationales
Utilize therapeutic communication techniques during interactions, such as unconditional acceptance, attention, respecting privacy and space requirements, encouraging verbalization of non-verbal cues, and giving positive feedback about actions.	Anxiety is reduced and opportunities for positive self-regard introduced.
Involve in activities that offer capability of success, i.e., occupational therapy, work assignment, or unit projects.	Opportunities for positive socialization and feedback from peers and staff are provided.
Involve in cognitive therapy groups to confront non-reality-based	Cognitive therapy or restructuring is a treatment modality that is

Nursing Interventions	Rationales
thinking about behaviors and self-expectations.	carried out either in one-to-one therapy or group situations. It stresses the connection between beliefs, thoughts, and action. The patient is taught to observe in what situations self-negating statements or images are created. Role playing, assertiveness training, and problem solving are also part of the training program.
Teach family/significant others about personality style (need to decrease anxiety and exert control over the environment), observe dynamics in relationship(s), and assist in identifying how changes will impact on family structure.	Changes in style of relating within a family or relationship will impact all members involved. Engaging significant others in identifying need and positive regard for change will facilitate the change process.

▶ NURSING DIAGNOSIS: *Anxiety*

Related To unconscious conflict about essential goals/values of life and need for control of everything in environment.

Defining Characteristics
- Restlessness/apprehensiveness
- Increased verbalization
- Inability to concentrate
- Physical symptoms of fight-or-flight response (dilated pupils, elevated pulse, elevated blood pressure, diarrhea, increased respirations)
- Appetite and sleep changes
- Lack of eye contact
- Self-focus

Patient Outcomes
Patient will
- employ coping mechanisms that allow interaction with the environment with minimal anxiety.
- experience an increase in psychological/physiological comfort.

Nursing Interventions	Rationales
Assess level of anxiety.	Ability to learn relaxation techniques and interventions that may be needed to help assist in decreasing anxiety are determined.
Stay with patient and present a calm demeanor. Provide empathy and speak in short, simple sentences.	This provides reassurance to patient and models for calming behavior.
Provide for time-out activity, encourage slow, deep breaths, and offer simple repetitive tasks.	Sensory stimulation is decreased and discomfort eased.
Administer anxiolytic agents if necessary to help patient maintain control.	If anxiety has reached severe or panic proportions, patient may need pharmacological help in regaining control and being able to attend to help being offered by staff.
Assist in identifying stressors that cause anxiety, behaviors that result, and methods for diminishing effect of stressors.	Identifying stressful events that cause anxiety, behavior that results, and positive coping mechanisms to decrease anxiety will help patients return to feelings of control over themselves and their emotions.

CONTINUITY OF CARE/DISCHARGE PLANNING
- Initiate one-to-one psychotherapy with cognitive-behavioral approach.
- Arrange for group psychotherapy on outpatient basis to encourage social support of positive changes in thinking and behavior.
- Encourage family therapy with goal that family will be able to support positive change.

BIBLIOGRAPHY
American Psychiatric Association (APA). (1994). *Diagnostic and statistical manual of mental disorders* (4th ed.). Washington, DC: APA.

Carpenito, L. (1992). *Nursing diagnosis: Application to clinical practice* (4th ed.). Philadelphia, PA: Lippincott.

Fortinash, K., & Holoday-Worret, P. (1991). *Psychiatric nursing care plans.* St. Louis, MO: Mosby-Year Book.

Jenike, M., Baer. L., & Minichiello, W. (1990). *Obsessive-compulsive disorders: Theory and management.* St. Louis, MO: Year-Book Medical.

Levenkron, S. (1991). *Treating and understanding crippling habits: Obsessive compulsive disorders.* New York: Warner.

North American Nursing Diagnosis Association (NANDA). (1992). *Nursing diagnosis: Definitions and classifications.* St. Louis, MO: NANDA.

Ryle, A. (1990). *Cognitive-analytic therapy: Active participation in change—A new integration in brief psychotherapy.* West Sussex, England: Wiley.

Townsend, M. (1991). *Nursing diagnosis in psychiatric nursing* (2nd ed.). Philadelphia, PA: Davis.

Wilson, H. & Kneisl, C. (1988). *Psychiatric nursing* (3rd ed.). Menlo Park, CA: Addison-Wesley.

APPENDIX : HUMAN RESPONSE PATTERNS OF THE NORTH AMERICAN NURSING DIAGNOSIS ASSOCIATION

Human Response Pattern	Definition
Choosing	To select between alternatives; the action of selecting or exercising preference in regard to a matter in which one is a free agent; to determine in favor of a course; to decide in accordance with inclinations
Communicating	To converse; to impart, confer, or transmit thoughts, feelings, or information, internally or externally, verbally or nonverbally
Exchanging	To give, relinquish, or lose something while receiving something in return; the substitution of one element for another, the reciprocal act of giving and receiving
Feeling	To experience a consciousness, sensation, apprehension, or sense; to be consciously or emotionally affected by a fact, event, or state
Knowing	To recognize or acknowledge a thing or a person; to be familiar with by experience or through information or report; to be cognizant of something through observation, inquiry, or information; to be conversant with a body of facts, principles, or methods of action; to understand
Moving	To change the place or position of a body or any member of the body; to put and/or keep in motion; to provoke an excretion or discharge; the urge to action or to do something; to take action
Perceiving	To apprehend with the mind; to become aware of by the senses; to apprehend what is not open or present to observation; to take in fully or adequately

Relating

To connect, establish a link between, or stand in some association to another thing, person, or place; to be borne or thrust in between things

Valuing

To be concerned about, to care; the worth or worthiness; the relative status of a thing or the estimate in which it is held, according to its real or supposed worth, usefulness, or importance; one's opinion of liking for person or thing; to equate in importance

INDEX